✝ AMERICAN LUNG ASSOCIATION®

7 Steps to a Smoke-Free Life

EDWIN B. FISHER JR., PH.D.
WITH TONI L. GOLDFARB

John Wiley & Sons, Inc.
New York   Chichester   Weinheim   Brisbane   Singapore   Toronto

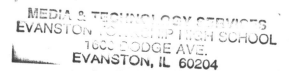

This book is dedicated to Frances V., in the hope it will provide the impetus for a longer, happier, healthier life; and to Edwin B. Fisher, who taught small lessons, like quitting smoking, large lessons, like living with enthusiasm and generosity, and the connections among them.

The information contained in this book is not intended to serve as a replacement for professional medical advice. Any use of the information in this book is at the reader's discretion. The author and publisher specifically disclaim any and all liability arising directly or indirectly from the use or application of any information contained in this book. A health care professional should be consulted regarding your specific situation.

Library of Congress Cataloging-in-Publication Data:
Fisher, Edwin B.
American Lung Association 7 steps to a smoke-free life/Edwin B. Fisher, Jr. with Toni L. Goldfarb.
p. cm.
Includes Index.
ISBN 0-471-24700-6 (pbk. alk. paper)
1. Smoking cessation programs. 2. Cigarette habit. I. Goldfarb, Toni L., II. American Lung Association III. Title.
HV5740.F525 1998
613.85—dc21   97-38826

Produced by LifeTime Media, Inc., New York, N.Y.
Printed in the United States of America
10 9 8 7 6 5 4 3

Contents

Part Three
PERFECTING THE NONSMOKING HABIT

Foreword

C. Everett Koop, M.D., Sc.D.

When I chose to become a physician more than half a century ago, my goal was to prolong life and to alleviate suffering. In my forty-year career I sought to do this one-on-one with my pediatric patients and their parents. As Surgeon General, I was able to do this by warning the American people about risks to their health, and educating them in ways to avoid premature death. As Surgeon General, I learned that we can prolong lives if we find the right way to get life-saving health messages to the people who need them. If you are one of the millions of smokers who needs help in becoming a nonsmoker, The American Lung Association's **7 Steps to a Smoke-Free Life** can be a real life-saver.

When you think about it, smoking is a strange habit: setting fire to something you then put in your mouth, breathing into your lungs the pungent smoke from chopped-up brown leaves, smoke that makes you and your house smell bad, smoke that will eventually shorten your life. It doesn't seem to be something that most thoughtful adults would choose to do.

And it isn't. Most adults don't want to smoke. And almost all adult smokers would like to quit. They know that smoking threatens to shorten their life. But they have real trouble quitting because they are addicted to the nicotine in tobacco. Right now about 25 percent of adult Americans smoke. But if our only adult smokers were those who really wanted to smoke, rather than those who smoke only because they are addicted, our smoking rate would fall to around 7 percent to 8 percent.

In human terms the cost is staggering. One thousand Americans die each day from the effects of smoking. According to careful calculations conducted by the Centers for Disease Control and Prevention, each cigarette steals seven minutes of life from a smoker. That adds up to five million lost years of life by American smokers each year.

There are today between 45 to 50 million nicotine addicts in the United States. All of them became addicted during the time when the tobacco industry lied to us by telling us nicotine was not addictive and that its tobacco products were not harmful. We all have an obligation to help the 15 to 20 million addicts who will die prematurely and poorly from a tobacco death.

Quitting smoking can be very difficult, but today smokers have a wider choice of smoking cessation tools available than ever before. **7 Steps to a Smoke-Free Life**, which can be used in conjunction with the growing number of nicotine replacement products and non-nicotine pharmaceuticals on the market, will make it easier than it used to be for today's smokers to become tomorrow's healthier ex-smokers.

Over the years I have worked with the American Lung Association to prevent young people from starting to smoke and helping those already hooked in breaking their addiction. The American Lung Association has more than ninety years of experience in fighting lung disease and promoting lung health. They have used that experience to develop their successful *Freedom From Smoking®* program, on which **7 Steps to a Smoke-Free Life** is based.

The author of this book, Edwin Fisher, Ph.D. has long been a key volunteer with the American Lung Association and a leader among smoking researchers. His experience in smoking cessation research and programs makes this book a rich source of knowledge and advice.

I wish you well as you embark on the challenging but very rewarding decision to quit for life.

Preface

Helping people quit smoking is central to the American Lung Association's mission to prevent lung disease and promote lung health. Smoking-related diseases claim more than 430,000 American lives each year.

Smoking is directly responsible for 87 percent of lung cancer cases and causes most cases of emphysema and chronic bronchitis. It is a major factor in coronary heart disease and stroke. Smoking by parents is also associated with a wide range of adverse effects in their children, including asthma flare-ups, increased frequency of cold and ear infections, and sudden infant death syndrome.

But the American Lung Association understands that just telling people smoking is harmful isn't enough to help them quit. As anyone reading this book probably knows, quitting smoking can be a very difficult process. For many people, breaking their addiction to nicotine can take many tries. That's why the American Lung Association provides a variety of materials and programs to help smokers in each stage of the quitting process. We help people quit in group settings, at work, online, and at home. We also have special programs for pregnant women, for African American smokers, and other diverse communities. And through the *Smoke-Free Class of 2000* and other educational programs, the American Lung Association is teaching children around the country about the dangers of tobacco, so they won't start smoking in the first place.

7 Steps to a Smoke-Free Life is based on the American Lung

Association's *Freedom From Smoking®* program, the gold standard of quit-smoking programs. Hundreds of thousands of ex-smokers will attest to *Freedom From Smoking's®* effectiveness. In an independent survey, the *Freedom From Smoking®* program was rated the most credible program on the market by more than 100 health maintenance organizations. The program is based on developing positive behavior change, building a support network, and focusing on effective relaxation techniques and strategies for maintaining your weight.

You can use **7 Steps to a Smoke-Free Life** to quit on your own, or use it in conjunction with one of the American Lung Association's smoking cessation clinics or other programs. The resources section at the back of this book lists local American Lung Association offices around the country. Call **1-800-LUNG-USA** to reach your local office, or visit us online at **http://www. lungusa.org** to find out more about our tobacco control programs and activities nationwide.

We hope **7 Steps to a Smoke-Free Life** helps you join the nation's 46 million ex-smokers.

Author's Note:
How I Quit Smoking

My father quit a three-pack-a-day Camel habit when I was about four years old. When I was about thirteen, my uncle died of lung cancer. Thus, I entered my teens thinking that smoking was a dangerous thing, that I would never do it. At about sixteen, I started smoking Camels, the unfiltered ones. I think I thought I was tough and independent but probably was only imitating my father. Anyway, I was sure I would never get hooked. After all, I was young and healthy, and I could quit before I "grew up."

As I approached January 1 of the year in which I would turn thirty, I was still smoking, now between one and a half and two packs a day. My closest friends said I still hadn't grown up but, at almost thirty, I knew I no longer qualified as a teenage smoker.

So, I did many of the things that we recommend in this book. I set a Quit Day and marshaled my energy in preparation for it. Using Do Power (see Step 4), I identified some predictable temptations and made plans for how I would cope with them. One that I remember was the pleasure of relaxing with one or two beers and a few cigarettes in the evening. For some reason, beer made me absolutely, dreadfully in need of a cigarette. However, the taste of brandy, which I also liked, seemed not to go with cigarettes at all. So, I bought myself a nice bottle of brandy and sipped it rather than beer when I relaxed in the evening. Now, brandy isn't for everyone, but the important point is to anticipate your temptation and make a plan for an alternative. Since I like the taste of brandy, I also gave myself a treat with this particular strategy.

I quit before the availability of nicotine replacement. I created my own by smoking pipes as a substitute. About a week after quitting, I was out on a Friday evening and forgot my pipe. So I returned to cigarettes for the weekend and quit again Monday morning. I consider myself lucky that this did not lead to a full relapse, as I had quit about ten times before—sometimes for as long as six months or a year—but had always slipped back. This time, however, I guess I was determined. Some of the credit for this should go to the chance remark of a colleague whose response to my most recent statement that I had quit had been "What, again?" Although it wasn't especially supportive, I think it did help me focus my attention on making this time different. And, as I will emphasize later in this book, quitting with determination is important.

I continued with the pipe for about six months after quitting and then decided that it, too, was more of a risk than I needed. Giving it up wasn't too difficult. I suspect this is like the experience of many people now who use nicotine gum or a nicotine patch for several months and then find them *relatively* easy to give up—nothing in this endeavor is easy!

That Monday that I quit again, after the Friday night semirelapse, was the Monday after the Super Bowl of January 1976. I haven't had a cigarette since. As I noted above, I stopped smoking pipes about four months after quitting cigarettes. About three years later, however, I began smoking cigars occasionally, as many as one a day while on vacation but usually two or three a month the rest of the year. About three years ago, a close friend became seriously ill with throat and lung cancer. She was a long-time smoker. At that time, not for health reasons but simply because I didn't want to give any more of my own energy to anything to do with tobacco, I gave up cigars, too. The only exception to this has been a few family gatherings at which my nephews have pushed me to join them in a cigar. I tried to persuade them that brandy tastes a lot better without the cigar smoke, but they can be very persuasive with their uncle!

In the last year, that friend and another have both died from smoking-related cancer. Over the years, as I became an active volunteer with the American Lung Association, my smoking friends often complimented me for not harassing them about their habit. "Ed, it's so great that, even though you're involved with the Lung Association and everything, you don't get on my case." Over the last several years, as I knew they were dying, I wondered often whether I should have gotten more on their case.

One of the points this book makes is that smoking is much more dangerous than people realize. It kills more people from cardiovascular disease—heart attacks and strokes—than from lung cancer! Although he quit smoking before he was 40, my father had his first stroke before he was 60. He lived another twenty years but we can only guess how much impact the smoking he was so proud to have given up had on the quality and the length of his life. I wonder, too, the impact it will have on mine, but I bolster and balance this every day with the medical knowledge that proves it was one of the best—albeit hardest—decisions of my life. This book is not meant to scare you into quitting. Rather, I hope it helps you figure out what you want to do about your smoking and to succeed at that. I think my father, my uncle, and my friends Judy and Bill would be pleased by that.

Introduction

Yes, You Can Quit Smoking... for Good!

You've thought about it a lot. Maybe you've tried once or twice before. But this time, you think you may really be ready. You feel you're definitely serious about wanting to quit smoking. Now! For good! And this book will show you how.

What's going to make the crucial difference for you is the expertise of the American Lung Association. The American Lung Association and its volunteer scientists, doctors, and citizens have been working for decades to understand why people smoke and how they quit. **7 Steps to a Smoke-Free Life** is based on the American Lung Association's respected *Freedom From Smoking®* program. Using this book, you'll be able to follow the program in your own home, without having to travel to group meetings.

If you've had a hard time trying to quit—and staying quit—on your own, the **7 Steps to a Smoke-Free Life** program is for you. It helps you figure out and enhance your own personal reasons to quit, helps you understand and cope with both the habit and addiction components of smoking, helps you make staying off cigarettes the priority it needs to be, and helps you plan effective ways to keep temptations to smoke from doing you in.

> "I thought quitting was just mind over matter. But it wasn't. The American Lung Association taught me how to quit. I learned how to keep my mind off cigarettes, how to keep from smoking when I'm with friends, and how to stay calm. You know what? This time I stopped for good." —Dennis, age 41

You're probably thinking, "Why should this approach work any better than the other quit-smoking programs I've tried that didn't help at all?" Here's why: The **7 Steps to a Smoke-Free Life** program treats you like the individual you are.

No two smokers are alike. This program helps you figure out why *you* smoke, and which people, places, and things trigger *your* unique urge to light up. It's individually designed for *you*. For example, you may have very personal reasons for smoking:

❏ You're under a lot of stress at work.
❏ All of your friends are smokers, so you can't escape it.
❏ Smoking helps you keep your weight down.
❏ You really have a strong addiction to cigarettes.
   You have trouble going an hour without one.
❏ You really enjoy smoking. It is pleasurable for you.
❏ You don't have the willpower to quit.
❏ Smoking helps you feel relaxed and positive.

Whatever your personal reasons for smoking may be, we'll help you to recognize them. Check out the Pack Track in Chapter 5, for example. It's the key to discovering where, when, and why *you* light up.

What Are the Obstacles?

In Chapter 3, you'll review the obstacles that have prevented you from quitting in the past. This time, you'll finally learn how to overcome each obstacle. You'll check off a list of roadblocks that are holding you back, and then one by one you'll learn how to clear them away.

For instance, what if you've never been able to quit smok-

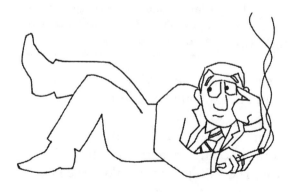

Me quit smoking? How?

ing for more than a few days? Your nicotine craving has always gnawed away at you, until you were forced to smoke "just one cigarette" to ease that discomfort. The **7 Steps to a Smoke-Free Life** program will give you some options for dealing with this. You may want to try nicotine fading (described in Chapter 7) to gradually reduce your nicotine cravings, before you quit altogether. That way, giving up cigarettes will be less difficult. Or you may want to try nicotine replacement—such as the patch or gum—to help you get used to not smoking before you have to give up nicotine entirely.

Once you've learned about these techniques and other ways to help yourself over the roadblocks, you're ready to select your own personalized quitting plan—your winning strategy—that's just right for *you* and your special needs. Then you can set that important date: *Your Quit Day.*

The Day You Actually Quit Smoking

It's going to be one of the most important days of your life. The step-by-step guide in Chapter 8 will set out specific day-by-day activities to prepare for your Quit Day. And Chapter 9 shows you exactly what to do on the big day, the day you actually quit smoking.

Of course, that's only the beginning. Many people face some tough times when they've stopped smoking, especially in the first week or two without cigarettes. But you'll be prepared for tough times. Whenever you want a cigarette, try the *Four D's.* You'll find them in Chapter 9. Or if you're feeling tense and irritable, use a simple Relaxercise that helps you stay calm without smoking. That's in Chapter 3. And we've got five more strategies to help you maintain your quit-smoking program, which you'll read about, too.

"Sure, this sounds good," you're thinking. "But what if I slip and smoke a cigarette or two? That's what's always happened before." Don't let this stop you. Millions of people who have quit

> **"A good thing about this program is that it showed me things I could do instead of smoking. That really helped me kick the habit."**
> **—Joanne, age 23**

smoking slip up. But in Chapter 10 of the **7 Steps to a Smoke-Free Life** program, you'll learn to treat a slip-up like an emergency, to keep a lapse from become a relapse. You'll be given the tools to handle the situation. You'll be armed with a nonsmoking strategy to last a lifetime.

> "Before this program, I had tried everything—hypnosis, acupuncture, even a plastic cigarette. Nothing really did the job. But The American Lung Association's 7 Step program is teaching me to change my life."—Bob, age 57

And, should the slip become a relapse, take heart. Most successful quitters relapsed a few times before they quit successfully. Chapter 12 helps you learn from your relapse and feel more confident about quitting again.

You're About to Become a Nonsmoker

Congratulations on taking this step toward quitting. You are on your way to doing one of the best things you can do for yourself and the people around you. You are now on your way to a smoke-free *you* and a smoke-free *life*. It will be a better life for you, and the people close to you.

PART ONE

Clearing the Air

The Facts

and Myths

about Your

Smoking Habit

CHAPTER 1

Getting to the Root of It: Why Do You Smoke?

If you had to choose *the one worst thing* about cigarette smoking, what would it be?

- ❑ Your doctor's warnings—and your own worries—that smoking can give you cancer, emphysema, strokes, or heart attacks
- ❑ The smoky smell that permeates your clothes, your furniture, your car, and all your belongings
- ❑ The overflowing ash trays throughout your house
- ❑ The increasing amount of money you have to spend to buy cigarettes
- ❑ The high dollar penalty you pay as a smoker when you purchase health and life insurance
- ❑ Difficulty finding places where you can smoke now that it's prohibited in so many public buildings, offices, and restaurants
- ❑ Your hoarse voice, frequent coughing, or shortness of breath
- ❑ The yellowish-brown stains on your hands and teeth
- ❑ The trouble you have smelling and tasting your food
- ❑ Guilt and frustration because you can't conquer your cravings for cigarettes, which makes you feel that cigarettes are controlling you
- ❑ Your spouse's complaints that inhaling your cigarette smoke is harming both your spouse's and your children's health

There certainly is a lot of bad stuff to choose from! So people must have many positive reasons to keep smoking. Psychologists call these **positive reinforcements**—another word for rewards. In scientific terms, a positive reinforcement is a pleasing consequence that makes someone more likely to repeat the behavior that led to it.

How Positive Reinforcement Works

Let's say you're feeling very tired at work after lunch. Your **response** is to smoke a cigarette. If the result of this behavior is that you feel less tired and more alert—**a positive reinforcement**—then you're more likely to smoke a cigarette again the next time you feel tired. In this example, not only is smoking reinforced by your feeling more alert, but each stimulus—sitting at your desk and realizing it's 3 in the afternoon—becomes associated with smoking. So, the next time you're feeling tired at your desk, whether it's 3 o'clock in the afternoon or 10 o'clock in the morning, you'll be likely to smoke a cigarette. And, the next time you're sitting at your desk at 3 p.m., even if you are *not* tired, you'll be likely to smoke a cigarette.

Of course, smoking isn't the only way to relieve fatigue. You could stand up and stretch, open a window and breathe deeply, or wash your face. But you chose to smoke a cigarette and it worked. In this instance, you *learned* that smoking a cigarette is a good way to relieve tiredness, and you're more likely to try smoking again the next time you're feeling tired. Behavioral scientists would say that you have learned to smoke in response to feeling tired.

If you've ever studied psychology, you might recall that this conditioning process is similar to the way a rat learns to run through a maze. If the rat is hungry (**stimulus**), it starts running around all the paths in the maze (**response**). By chance, the rat finally runs down the path that has a piece of cheese at the end (**positive reinforcement**). The rat eats the cheese and feels better. After this stimulus-response-reinforcement sequence is repeated a few times, we'd say the rat has learned the maze, and it's very likely to follow the correct path whenever it's put in the maze.

The Rewards of Smoking

What does all this have to do with smoking? Plenty! Researchers have found that cigarette smoking is a behavior that people repeat again and again, because it provides so many positive reinforcements. Unlike the rat that gets cheese only in a maze, smokers get a lot of reinforcement from their cigarettes and these reinforcers become associated with many circumstances in everyday life. For example, ask yourself why you smoke, and you're likely to name many positive reinforcements, such as:

- ❑ Smoking relaxes me.
- ❑ Cigarettes perk me up and make me feel energized.
- ❑ Smoking helps to relieve my feelings of stress and anger.
- ❑ Smoking keeps me from slowing down.
- ❑ Smoking with friends adds to my social enjoyment.
- ❑ Smoking keeps me occupied when I'm waiting in line, stuck in traffic, or just feeling bored.
- ❑ And talking on the phone, finishing a meal, or having a cup of coffee just seem to need a cigarette to go with them.

These rewards of smoking go a long way toward minimizing the negative consequences, and an even longer way toward ensuring that the act of smoking will be repeated again and again, until it becomes a **habit** so well ingrained you do it without even thinking about it.

Let's do the math together. If you smoke a pack a day, that's 20 cigarettes every day, 140 cigarettes each week, about 600 each month, and over 7,000 in just one year. Multiply that by the number of years *you* have been smoking. On average, you inhale seven times with each cigarette. During a twenty-year period, it's estimated that the average pack-a-day smoker inhales cigarette smoke more than *1 million times.* Is it any wonder that the smoking habit is so hard to break?

HOW MANY CIGARETTES HAVE YOU SMOKED?

20	cigarettes a day
x 365	days per year
7,300	cigarettes each year
x 20	years smoked
146,000	cigarettes smoked in a lifetime

"I think I smoked to calm down. My job can be stressful at times, and I used to smoke to relax."
—Michele, age 31

But smoking isn't just a habit—*it's both a habit and an addiction.* The nicotine in cigarettes is a powerful addictive drug that makes smokers feel good. Each time you smoke, the positive biological effects of nicotine are added to all the other positive rewards of smoking, which makes the smoking habit even stronger.

What Nicotine Does

Nicotine is a pretty remarkable drug. It works in many different situations. If you're feeling tense, nicotine relaxes you. If you're feeling drowsy, nicotine increases your alertness. If you're feeling sad, it elevates your mood. If you're feeling hungry, it calms your hunger pangs.

What's really impressive is that a smoker can get all of these benefits, even though they may seem contradictory. That's why skillful smokers have their first cigarette of the day to get going when they get up in the morning, and their last of the day to calm down before they turn out the light to go to sleep at night.

One way nicotine does all this is by altering chemicals in the brain. Chemicals that carry messages from one nerve to another play important roles in our mood and feeling alert. In smokers who have gotten used to it, nicotine helps keep those brain chemicals in the right balance to feel happy and ready to meet the day.

So in a lot of ways, nicotine is an amazing drug. And the cigarette is a wonderful way to get nicotine. The "uptake" of nicotine is very quick. It takes just seven seconds for nicotine to go from your lips to your lungs, and then to a major artery that takes it right up to your brain.

And the "clearance time" of nicotine is quick, too—it leaves your body pretty quickly. When you've had too much, you get over it in an hour or so. It's not like a hangover that lasts into the next day. So, with its quick uptake to the brain and quick clearance time, smokers can adjust their nicotine levels to get whatever effect they want: mood elevating, anxiety lowering, stimulating.

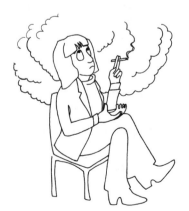

Yes, nicotine really is pretty remarkable. And smokers surely aren't crazy to want to smoke. It's just unfortunate that the way we get nicotine—tobacco cigarettes—kills so many of us.

If you smoke a pack a day, you inhale smoke about 60,000 times in one year.

Other Effects of Nicotine

In addition to its psychological effects, nicotine affects almost every system in the body. Take just a puff or two on a cigarette, and your heart beats faster, your pulse quickens, your veins constrict, your blood pressure increases. Your adrenal glands pump out epinephrine (adrenaline) that increases your heart rate, relaxes many of your smooth muscles, and raises your metabolic rate. Even the electrical activity in your brain changes.

These are powerful biological effects. Indeed, nicotine is a very powerful drug. It's one of the most toxic of all drugs, comparable to cyanide. Take enough nicotine and it can kill you. But the amount of nicotine in a single cigarette is only 8 to 9 milligrams on average, a very small amount. (A milligram is one-thousandth of a gram; it would take over 28,000 milligrams to make just one ounce.)

The amount of nicotine that smokers inhale from each cigarette is even smaller. Most popular brands of cigarettes deliver less than 1.5 milligrams per cigarette. This amount may be somewhat higher or lower for each smoker, depending on how deeply you puff and how many puffs you take from each cigarette.

But nicotine is so potent that even this minuscule dose causes significant changes in the functioning of numerous organs and systems in your body. When people first take up smoking, these physiological changes feel extremely unpleasant. Beginning smokers typically experience nausea, dizziness, headache, stomach distress, coughing, and other uncomfortable symptoms. But people who continue to smoke soon develop a tolerance to these symptoms, until most symptoms become unnoticeable.

How Tolerance Develops

Tolerance is a term used to describe an important feature of addiction. Tolerance has developed when, after the repeated administration of a drug (in this case, nicotine), a given dose of the drug produces a decreased effect. Or conversely, tolerance has developed when increasingly larger doses must be administered to obtain the effects observed with the original dose.

What does this mean for a smoker? The small dose of nicotine delivered by several puffs on a cigarette may make people feel ill the first few times they try smoking. But after they've been smoking for a week or so (repeated "self-administration" of nicotine), several puffs and even an entire cigarette no longer have that effect. Now they'll feel ill only if, let's say, they smoke several cigarettes one after another (a larger dose).

More important, tolerance to the unpleasant physiological effects of nicotine permits the smoker to focus on nicotine's pleasurable physiological effects. Many smokers don't realize that nicotine's effects on the heart, the nervous system, and the endocrine system are significant contributors to the relaxation, alertness, stress relief, and other good feelings they experience while smoking. This combination of physiological and psychological effects provides so much positive reinforcement that smoking quickly becomes an established habit.

Physical and Psychological Dependence

As the term *tolerance* implies, a smoker actually becomes accustomed to having a certain level of nicotine in his or her body. In fact, research studies have shown that, without consciously realizing it, smokers regulate the number of cigarettes they smoke in order to maintain their own personally preferred level of nicotine. For example, smokers who are given a very high nicotine cigarette will puff less often than usual, so they don't take in more nicotine than their preferred amount. Similarly, with a low nicotine cigarette, the smoker will take more puffs than usual, in order to get that preferred amount of nicotine.

Of course, when no cigarettes are smoked for a while—for example, when someone is trying to quit smoking—the smoker doesn't get any nicotine. Now it's the *lack* of nicotine that produces unpleasant physiological symptoms in the body. Medically, these symptoms are called *withdrawal effects.*

To relieve these physical withdrawal effects, many smokers must continue to take in their usual amount of nicotine. This is a sign of **physical dependence** on nicotine. Doctors define physical dependence as a change in the body's functioning that is produced by repeated administration of a drug, such that continued doses of the drug are needed to prevent withdrawal symptoms.

But that's not all. Smokers also become accustomed to the psychological effects of smoking. After the smoking habit is established, the smoker needs to smoke in order to feel "normal." In other words, the effects produced by nicotine, and the behaviors associated with smoking, become necessary to maintain the person's optimal state of well-being. This condition is referred to as **psychological dependence**.

At the extreme, many smokers who run out of cigarettes or are unable to smoke, such as in a movie theater, then become totally preoccupied by thoughts of having a cigarette. It's like the old advertising slogan "I'd walk a mile for a *Camel.*" This behavior is often referred to as **compulsive drug use**.

Is Smoking an Addiction?

Physiological and physical dependence, withdrawal, and compulsive drug use are the defining characteristics of **drug addiction**. Does that mean smoking is an addiction to nicotine?

Certainly the smoking habit meets many of the criteria needed to qualify as an addiction, including:

1. A highly controlled or compulsive pattern of drug use: The experienced smoker has lots of smoking patterns that, if broken, are disturbing. And many would walk that mile for a *Camel.*

2. Psychoactive or mood-altering effects involved in the pattern of drug taking: These are the mood-altering, anxiety-reducing, and stimulating effects we noted earlier.

3. Drug functioning as a reinforcer to strengthen behavior and lead to further drug ingestion: It's the nicotine that keeps people smoking—ginseng or herbal cigarettes just don't measure up!

Using these criteria, the 1988 U.S. Surgeon General's Report on smoking made several major conclusions:

▶ Cigarettes and other forms of tobacco are addicting.

▶ Nicotine is the drug in tobacco that causes addiction.

▶ The pharmacological and behavioral processes that determine tobacco addiction are similar to those that determine addiction to drugs such as heroin and cocaine.

All smokers show signs of physical and psychological dependence on nicotine. Their bodies crave nicotine, and they will smoke until their bodies have taken in a certain level of nicotine. Thus, addiction is more a matter of degree. It's not if you are addicted, but *how addicted* you are. However, this doesn't mean it's impossible to quit. It simply takes a different kind of strategy, which you'll discover in the 7 Steps.

Triggering the Habit

It's important to remember that smoking is both a habit and an addiction. There are many times when you tell yourself you're going to have a cigarette. But often, the smoking you do is just out of habit.

Habits are affected by your environment. Something you see or do in your daily life—a cue or a trigger—gets them going. Triggers are the stimuli associated with smoking and its reinforcers, as we mentioned earlier.

What are smoking triggers? Think back to when you had just started to smoke. At first your only positive reinforcement might have been social acceptance from your friends: "They'll think I'm 'cool' if I smoke." That reward helped to counter the initial negative consequences—nausea, bad taste in your mouth, tearing eyes, and burning throat. The more you smoked, the less bothered you were by the physical discomforts. And almost without realizing it, you quickly began to enjoy smoking for many new reasons:

❑   You often smoked during the happy times you spent with friends. As a result, you're now likely to smoke whenever you want to feel happier.

❑   You found that you ate less when you smoked, and that's helped you to control your weight. As a result, you now light a cigarette whenever you feel hungry but don't want to eat. You may even smoke between courses at a meal.

❑   Phone calls from your family members may sometimes be stressful. When they call, you frequently light up a cigarette to help yourself stay calm. Now you find yourself reaching for a smoke whenever you make a phone call or answer the phone, no matter who's on the line.

❑   If you're alone and have nothing to do, you tend to think about your worries and anxieties. You've found that smoking relaxes you and makes you feel happier. Cigarettes have become like "a friend" to you. In fact, you realize that you smoke the most when no friends are around and you're feeling lonely, worried, sad, or just bored.

People often say cigarettes are a "crutch" because smokers lean on their cigarettes for help in so many situations—being with friends, eating, talking on the phone, or just feeling bored. Triggers can be any number of things, bad and good. And different smokers have different triggers. You may connect a cigarette so strongly with a particular activity that you'd have trouble carrying out that activity without a cigarette.

For instance, some smokers always smoke when they have a cup of coffee. Other smokers can't go to sleep until they've had that last cigarette of the night. Nicotine addiction is the reason. The physiological effects of nicotine combine with the effects of your morning coffee to give you the extra stimulation you need to get going. Similarly, the negative feelings that nicotine counteracts (feeling sad, anxious, stressed out) all evoke strong urges for a cigarette. So you have a cigarette at bedtime, you feel more relaxed, and you're able to fall asleep.

THE THREE BIG REASONS FOR SMOKING

1. Nicotine is a powerful reinforcer.

2. The act of smoking offers many positive reinforcements.

3. The reinforcement becomes associated with many cues and activities in daily life.

So, smoking becomes tied to many satisfactions each day.

As you can see, triggers tend to expand and make new connections. By the time most smokers have bought this book, they may feel that almost everything they do has become a trigger for smoking. This may be true, but as you will see later, an important part of getting ready to quit is breaking up some of your strongest smoking triggers.

Smoking Is More Than Just Puffing

The process of smoking also involves buying cigarettes, removing each cigarette from the pack, lighting it, locating and handling an ashtray, blowing the smoke out of your mouth and nose, watching the smoke rise in the air, feeling the cigarette in your hand, flicking off the ashes, stubbing it out when you're finished, among many other things. In a sense, these too become

> "I smoked at all my work breaks, and used to smoke as many cigarettes as I could before I had to go back to work."
> —Anastazia, age 42

triggers—the sight of the ashtray, for example.

The steps in smoking—from pouring the cup of coffee to lighting up, to stubbing it out when done—all of these become woven into a highly organized pattern that's repeated each time you smoke. Each individual action becomes reinforcing through its connection to the others in the pattern, and the eventual nicotine to which they lead. The entire array of behaviors soon takes its place as an integral part of your daily life.

Just as a person who's recently retired from a job complains that "I don't know what to do with myself," it's no wonder that people who try to quit smoking complain that "Smoking is almost constantly on my mind," and worry that they'll be unable to do without it. The cues and triggers are everywhere!

Your own personal smoking triggers—how often they occur and how strong they are—are what determine your smoking habit pattern.

Numerous research studies indicate that the single most helpful thing you can do to break the smoking habit is to take it off automatic pilot—to stop and notice your smoking triggers. As you'll see in Chapter 5, identifying and counteracting those triggers is an important key to quitting smoking.

Learning More about Why You Smoke

If you think you are ready to start taking immediate steps toward quitting, or if you'd like a good way to understand your own reasons for smoking, this next section is especially for you. If neither of these fit you right now, turn to Chapter 2 to learn more about how smoking affects your body and what you can do about it. You'll learn more about the Pack Track described here when you are ready to begin your quitting program.

If You Want to Start Now

If you just throw your cigarettes away and say, "I'm going to quit right now," the smoking triggers in your life are likely to overwhelm you. You'll be more likely to succeed if you identify your triggers *before* you quit and make plans to cope with them. To help you do this, the American Lung Association has designed a method called "Pack Track," which you'll read about in more detail in Part Two of this book.

But if you'd like to get a head start on quitting right away, tear out one of the Pack Track cards on page 59. You'll notice that the card is the same size as your cigarette pack. Attach the card to a full pack of cigarettes with a rubber band or put it inside the cellophane. Every time you take a cigarette from the pack, write down the time, the mood you're in, and how much you want that cigarette.

TRACK YOUR MOODS

If you're in a **good** mood, put a check mark under the smiling face.

If you're in a **bad** mood, check the sad face.

If you feel **in-between**, check the middle face.

If you **really** want that cigarette, check "YES." (capital letters)

If you want it but **not a lot**, check "yes." (small letters)

If it's **no big deal**, check "???"

DATE:						
No.	Time	???	yes	YES	😊	😐 😞
1						
2						
3						
4						
5						
6						
7						
8						
9						
10	© AMERICAN LUNG ASSOCIATION, 1993					

After you've finished the entire package of cigarettes, read over your Pack Track card and ask yourself some important questions:

❑ Did you smoke more often than you thought, or less often?

❑ What was the mood that showed up most often on your cards?

❑ How often was your need for a cigarette very high?

Your answers will help you identify the places, times, moods, and conditions that trigger your need to smoke. You may be surprised by what you learn. You can continue to use the Pack Track cards while you read through the next sections of the book. When you come to Part Two, you'll find out how to make Pack Track a part of your **7 Step** smoking cessation program.

CHAPTER 2

The Costs of Smoking— and the Benefits of Quitting

If you've bought this book and read this far, you know that smoking is harmful to your health. It's no secret—The Surgeon General's Warning is clearly marked on every pack of cigarettes. Over 40,000 careful studies have proven that smoking causes disease and death. Every medical and health agency agrees, and numerous surveys have shown that most Americans do realize smoking is risky. Just how great the risks are is what this chapter will address.

SURGEON GENERAL'S WARNING: Smoking Causes Lung Cancer, Heart Disease, Emphysema, And May Complicate Pregnancy

The American Lung Association has found that having a bit more clarity about the dangers of smoking and recognizing your personal risks in addition to the general risk factors can help you develop the determination to quit. The objective of this chapter isn't to depress you, but to increase your motivation. You *can* quit, and the benefits of quitting will begin sooner than you think.

Smoking Must Be Singled Out

When urged to quit smoking, people often say, "Well, I don't have too many other vices." They've failed to grasp that smoking deserves to be singled out. The enormous impact of smoking dwarfs the effects of most other risks.

Here are the facts:

▶ Smoking is the greatest source of preventable death in our society.

▶ Smoking accounts for 1 out of every 6 or 7 (or more than 400,000) deaths each year in the United States.

▶ Every year, more Americans die from smoking-related diseases than from AIDS, drug abuse, car accidents,and murder—combined.

▶ Children of smokers are exposed to second hand smoke, which significantly increases their risk of developing asthma, ear infec tions, pneumonia, and bronchitis.

▶ 87 percent of all lung cancer cases are caused by smoking.

▶ One out of every two long-term smokers die because of smoking.

▶ Smokers die on average 6 to 8 years younger than non-smokers do.

Here's another fact you may not know: Smoking kills more people through heart disease than through lung cancer. And although many women are worried about breast cancer, studies show that lung cancer now kills more women than breast cancer. Since 1950, there has been a 500 percent increase in female lung cancer deaths in the United States. In fact, lung cancer now surpasses breast cancer as the leading cause of cancer deaths in American women.

"ANNA"

When she was just a little girl, Anna used to sit by her mother and light her cigarettes. Striking the matches made her feel grownup, and it was only natural that Anna would soon emulate the woman she most admired and take up smoking herself. Like others in her generation, Anna had no idea that smoking was harmful. By the time health warnings were issued, she was hooked....

The Effects of Smoke in Your Body

Cigarette ads always picture smiling, active people in romantic or "fun" situations. None of the smokers is ever seen coughing or stopping to catch their breath during the lively sports events or lights-down-low dinners the tobacco advertisers often portray.

The real picture of smoking isn't very pretty. Have you ever seen a photograph of a smoker's lungs? Lungs that haven't been exposed to cigarette smoke and other pollutants have a healthy pink color, but smokers' lungs are a sickly, tar-black color.

"ANNA"

Anna wasn't too worried about her lungs. She never smoked more than a pack a day, nor had any early warnings—smoker's cough or shortness of breath—to tell her she was damaging her health.

If you're not sure how bad that looks, you might want to try the old test you probably did as a teenager. Take a clean white tissue and exhale several puffs of cigarette smoke directly through it. The gunky discoloration that you see is just like the gunk in a smoker's lungs. Only multiply that tissue mess one million times— that's the estimated number of puffs a pack-a-day smoker takes over a twenty-year period.

If blowing smoke through a tissue isn't for you, try this imaging device. Create a mental image of cancer cells destroying your lungs, mouth, throat, esophagus, gastrointestinal tract, and urinary tract. If you're a woman, add your cervix. Tobacco use has been linked to cancers of these and other vital organs.

"ANNA"

Anna was distressed when her weight suddenly dropped by thirty pounds. Food smelled bad and tasted worse to her. Day and night, she felt an itch to cough that was never relieved. She went to the doctor, who ordered a chest X-ray. The X-ray showed a mass in her upper right lung, and a biopsy confirmed her fears. It was small-cell lung cancer, a particularly aggressive type that can rarely be cured by surgery.

Recent statistics show that the vast majority of lung cancers— about 87 percent—are caused by smoking. What's worse, the disease is often symptomless in the early stages. Thus, when the disease is discovered it's often so far advanced that a cure is impossible. While these facts may have you thinking, "Why bother? The damage has already been done," then quickly read on to some of the more heartening facts.

So If I Quit Now, Will I Live Longer?

Did you know that people who quit smoking live longer than people who continue to smoke? After fifteen years off cigarettes, the risk of death for ex-smokers returns to nearly the level of people who have never smoked. Male smokers who quit between ages 35 to 39 add an average of five years to their lives. Female quitters in this age group add three years to their lives. These are averages—for some people, it's a lot more years.

If you're thinking that the earlier facts about lung disease don't apply to you, as your family has no history of lung cancers, it's important to consider the following: It's a surprisingly overlooked fact that even more people die from **heart disease** associated with smoking than from smoking-related cancers. In patients with **diabetes**, a condition which often leads to heart disease, smoking further increases heart and stroke risks.

Tobacco use is also associated with other diabetic complications, including nervous system damage (neuropathy) and **blindness** caused by damage to the retinas of the eyes (retinopathy). Blindness due to age-related macular degeneration is also more common among diabetics and nondiabetics who smoke. So, if either heart disease or diabetes is part of your family's medical history, the facts about the dangers of smoking are just as applicable to you.

The Sad Truth about the Marlboro Man and Virginia Slims Woman

Prematurely aged, wrinkled skin, and even baldness are also common in men and women who smoke. In addition, female smokers have an increased risk of osteoporosis, the bone loss that causes stooped posture and hip fractures. Male impotence—inability to have an erection—is another common but often "unmentioned" side effect of smoking, especially in smokers who also have diabetes. Studies have shown that, in smokers, blood flow to the penis is reduced, which diminishes erections. Many male smokers also have lowered sperm counts and decreased fertility. This is all especially ironic, considering that tobacco ads often picture macho men and sexy women in romantic situations.

> **"Quitting smoking is one of the best things that you can do for yourself. You'll feel better, your health will improve, and you'll live longer. It's not easy, but if you really want to quit, you can do it."**
> **—Kimberly, age 38**

Fortunately, some of these conditions are reversible. For example, one study of twenty impotent heavy smokers found that after quitting for just six weeks, seven men (35%) were again able to have erections. If you're a man who's having problems in bed, isn't this a good reason to forget about smoking?

In addition to a rejuvenated sex life, there are other *immediate* benefits to quitting: your body will start to change for the better within the first twenty minutes after you stop smoking. The tiny hair-like cilia inside your nasal passages immediately start to sweep away germs and pollutants. Many other systems in the body also show quick changes. Here's what you can expect:

WHEN SMOKERS QUIT

Within twenty minutes of smoking that last cigarette, the body begins a series of changes

AT 20 MINUTES AFTER QUITTING
- ▶ Blood pressure decreases
- ▶ Pulse rate drops
- ▶ Body temperature of hands and feet increases

AT 8 HOURS
- ▶ Carbon monoxide level in blood drops to normal
- ▶ Oxygen level in blood increases to normal

AT 24 HOURS
- ▶ Chance of a heart attack decreases

AT 48 HOURS
- ▶ Nerve endings start regrowing
- ▶ Ability to smell and taste is enhanced

In addition to these biological benefits, you'll just feel better. Even before all your urges for cigarettes have ended, you'll find your energy going up, and you'll be able to do more of the things you enjoy. You'll also have more money in your pockets to help you do those things.

You'll look better immediately, because toxic gases will no longer make your eyes water, or irritate your nose and throat. And, you'll look better in the long run as you wrinkle less, keep more hair, and feel great on your way to the gym, the newest play or restaurant, to visit your children—or your grandchildren! It beats emphysema, smoker's cough, bronchitis, chest pain, and wrinkles, doesn't it?

Symptoms of Emphysema

Cigarette smoking is a primary culprit in **chronic obstructive pulmonary disease (COPD)**, which is the fourth-ranking cause of death in the United States (after heart attacks, cancers, and stroke). Nearly 16 million Americans have COPD. Smoking accounts for 82 percent of all deaths from this disease.

COPD isn't a pretty picture. **Emphysema**, one common form of COPD, develops over many years of smoking-related damage to lung tissues. The walls between the tiniest air sacs within the lungs break down. Elasticity of the lung tissue is lost, and the lungs become distended, so they can't expand and contract normally. As emphysema progresses, the effort needed to breathe increases and, ultimately, each breath becomes a chore. Because the lungs and the heart have to work harder to get enough oxygen into the bloodstream, continuous administration of oxygen is needed. Meanwhile, the patient grows progressively weaker due to shortness of breath, until even minor physical activity is impossible.

What does this feel like? If you have ever been at the top of a very high mountain, where the air is thin, you know the sensation. Even climbing a few steps or picking up a bundle causes alarming huffing, puffing, and physical exhaustion. Victims of emphysema live with this problem every minute of the day.

"Smoker's Cough" and Chronic Bronchitis

"Smoker's cough"—that heavy chest cough so common in long-term tobacco users—is also a warning sign of **chronic bronchitis**, another form of COPD.

The bronchi are the main air passages of the lungs. Inflammation of the mucous membrane that lines the bronchi is called **bronchitis**. It's usually caused by a virus infection. The major symptoms are a deep cough that brings up heavy phlegm from your lungs, wheezing, breathlessness, and fever.

People who have a healthy heart and healthy lungs usually recover from bronchitis in just a few days. But in smokers, the bronchial inflammation persists and worsens, causing narrowing and obstruction of the tiny bronchioles that branch off the bronchi. The first symptom of this **chronic bronchitis** is a morning cough that brings up heavy phlegm. Smokers often think this is just their "normal" smoker's cough, but the amount of phlegm increases and soon coughing occurs throughout the day. A daily productive cough is *not* normal!

In the later stages, breathlessness and wheezing become so bad that medication and supplementary oxygen are needed to sustain breathing. Susceptibility to bronchial infections increases and can eventually lead to pneumonia, emphysema, and even death.

What's the most effective treatment? You guessed it: *quitting smoking.*

The Continuing Benefits of Quitting

Yes, there's more to come. Once you've quit, your body systems and your overall health continue to improve throughout the first year you're off cigarettes. Following are just some of the benefits:

THE FIRST YEAR AFTER QUITTING

*After you quit smoking, the body begins
a series of changes that continues for years.*

AT 2 WEEKS TO 3 MONTHS
- ▶ Circulation improves.
- ▶ Walking becomes easier.
- ▶ Lung function increases.

1 TO 9 MONTHS
- ▶ Coughing, sinus congestion, fatigue, shortness of breath decrease.

1 YEAR
- ▶ Excess risk of coronary heart disease is decreased to half that of a smoker.

"ANNA"

So far, Anna's determination and medical care have paid off. The initial treatments sent her cancer into remission. Her appetite and strength came back, and after six months, she returned to the work she loves.

On her Saturdays off, Anna can often be found at her doctor's office, receiving maintenance treatment. By now, the ordeal has almost become routine. First, she receives two shots of nausea-preventing medicine. Chemotherapy follows fifteen minutes later. The powerful tumor-killing drugs used to be injected into veins in her arm, but those veins have now collapsed. The doctor surgically implanted a tiny pump beneath her skin to deliver medication directly into a large vein that empties blood into the heart. He kneads her chest to position the pump to receive three injections. As he prods, Anna closes her eyes and swallows hard.

In addition, you'll probably notice many other changes. For example, chronic irritation of the larynx is reduced, so your speaking voice may improve. Shortness of breath and coughing will occur much less often. You'll probably have fewer colds. And if you suffer from asthma, the frequency and severity of your asthma episodes will greatly decrease. The same holds true for someone in your household who has asthma but no longer has to breathe your "passive" smoke. Your peripheral and night vision may also improve, so you'll drive more safely, especially at night.

WHAT IF YOU'RE ALREADY SICK?

What if you already have a smoking-related illness? You'll be glad to know that the benefits of quitting smoking also apply to people who are currently sick:

For people with . . .   **Quitting smoking . . .**

HEART DISEASE ⟶ Reduces the risk of repeat heart attacks and death from heart disease by 50 percent or more.

PERIPHERAL ARTERY DISEASE ⟶ Improves ability to exercise (poor circulation to the legs) and increases overall survival.

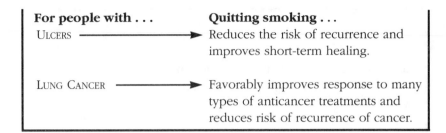

For people with . . .	Quitting smoking . . .
ULCERS ⟶	Reduces the risk of recurrence and improves short-term healing.
LUNG CANCER ⟶	Favorably improves response to many types of anticancer treatments and reduces risk of recurrence of cancer.

Discounting the Risks

Why do people discount so many of the well-known smoking risks? For one thing, almost every smoker has an Uncle Pete or Aunt Jane who "smoked like a chimney" and still lived to a ripe old age. Focusing on the exceptions makes it easier to forget that about half of all regular cigarette smokers will eventually be killed as a result of this habit. And even though Pete and Jane looked healthy, they had unseen damage to the delicate tissues in the throat, lungs, and other organs. Think back: they did cough a lot didn't they? In addition, they may have had a lot of other problems that no one ever thought were related to smoking—such as heart disease, diabetic complications, stroke, and even impotence. So, if you have the gene pool that's going to let you live to a ripe old age like Uncle Peter or Aunt Jane, why not live to a hearty ripe old age—far more feasible if you've quit smoking.

What About Secondhand Smoke?

Even people who don't smoke are often exposed to other people who smoke. Inhaling someone else's cigarette smoke is called **passive smoking** or **involuntary smoking**. It is a proven health hazard to nonsmokers, and it's not easy to avoid, because about one in four people smoke.

Did you know that **secondhand smoke**—the smoke breathed out by smokers and the smoke from the burning end of a cigarette, cigar, or pipe—has twice as much nicotine, and five times the carbon monoxide, as the smoke you inhale?

The U.S. Environmental Protection Agency lists secondhand smoke as a Group A carcinogen, a rating used only for substances proven to cause cancer in humans. In fact, the risk of lung cancer is about 30 percent higher for non-smoking wives of smokers than it is for nonsmoking wives of nonsmokers.

The health effects of second-hand smoke are controversial. Estimates range from about 5,000 to about 60,000 deaths a year—many fewer than the 400,000 attributed to regular smoking, but still far too many. Exposure to secondhand smoke can cause nonsmokers to cough, sneeze, and suffer eye irritations.

Secondhand Smoke and Children

Secondhand smoke poses special dangers to children. Well-documented research has shown that:

A study of 11,534 elementary school students throughout the United States and Canada conducted by researchers at the Boston University School of Medicine found that children exposed to secondhand smoke at home were 70 percent more likely to have wheezing with colds, 60 percent more likely to go to the emergency room for wheezing, and 40 percent more likely to have persistent wheezing compared with kids in homes without secondhand smoke.

Approximately half of all children studied were exposed to secondhand smoke at home at the time of the study. About 25 percent lived in homes with two or more smokers, and 13 percent were in homes where more than thirty cigarettes were smoked every day.

▶ Babies of smokers are more prone to pneumonia and bronchitis in the first year of life than are babies of nonsmokers.
▶ Children who breathe secondhand smoke have more ear infections, pneumonia, bronchitis, and lung diseases, and are more likely to develop asthma.
▶ Smoke in the home can worsen symptoms in asthmatic children and even trigger asthmatic attacks in young and adult nonsmokers.

Studies have also shown that children of smokers are more likely to start smoking themselves than are children of nonsmokers.

Smoking and Pregnancy

When a smoker becomes pregnant, her baby involuntarily becomes a passive smoker. The nicotine, carbon monoxide, and other poisons in tobacco smoke pass into the placenta that carries blood and nutrients from the mother's body directly into the baby's body. These poisons compete for space in the bloodstream with the food and oxygen the baby needs.

The major result is an increased risk of both miscarriage and low birth weight. A small, low-weight baby is often sick with many health problems. Smaller babies are more likely to need special care and to stay longer in the hospital.

Studies have also shown that if a woman's partner smokes near her during her pregnancy, this also raises the risk of delivering a baby that weighs too little and has health problems.

Now the Good News: Unique First-Year Quitting Benefits for Women

Smoking poses special risks for women, but women also derive unique benefits if they quit smoking. For example, compared to nonsmokers, it takes female smokers longer to get pregnant. However, women who quit smoking before trying to get pregnant have just as good a chance of becoming pregnant as women who have never smoked.

It takes female smokers longer to get pregnant.

Similarly, women who stop smoking before becoming pregnant or during their first trimester of pregnancy reduce their risk of having a low-birth-weight baby. If they continue not to smoke during the remainder of pregnancy, their risk of low birth-weight is as low as that of women who have never smoked.

In fact, a 1990 report from the U.S. Surgeon General concluded that, if all women quit smoking during pregnancy, about 5 percent of deaths among newborn infants could be prevented. Thanks to stepped-up education campaigns by the media, doctors, and health groups such as the American Lung Association, this important news is reaching women. It's now estimated that about 30 percent of women who are cigarette smokers quit after learning they are pregnant. Unfortunately, about 33 percent of pregnant women in the United States still smoke throughout pregnancy. If this applies to you—or someone close to you who is pregnant—quitting smoking should be your highest priority.

"ANNA"

When she passes young women who are smoking while she walks down the street, they don't give Anna a second glance. With her energetic walk and attractive wig, they couldn't guess what she's been through. But Anna would like them to know what she's experienced. "I want to tell them 'Stop. It's no good for you. Stop smoking before it's too late.' "

So, Can I Have a Cigar When the Baby's Born?

Tobacco advertisers have done a good job promoting cigars as a safe, pleasurable, sexy alternative to cigarettes. This has spawned a fad of "cigar bars" and even magazines devoted to cigar smoking and cigar paraphernalia such as humidors and clippers. Ad campaigns featuring celebrities—including female celebrities—who smoke cigars attempt to create a glamorous aura around smoking, which is still unhealthy and too often deadly.

DID DAD'S SPERM GO UP IN SMOKE? Several research studies have found that men who smoke suffer damage to their sperm—lower sperm count and difficulties in fertilization. Babies produced from those damaged sperm can have an increased risk of childhood cancers, including acute leukemia and lymphoma. Researchers say as many as 15% of all childhood cancers might be linked to smoking by fathers.

Many cigar smokers light up on special occasions, or smoke only two to three cigars a day. Because they smoke so few, they assume there are few health hazards. Wrong! A recent report notes that one large cigar may contain as much tobacco as a whole pack of cigarettes. And a smoker may spend up to an hour smoking a single large cigar, often in the presence of other smokers puffing on their own large cigars. Just breathing the air is a health hazard under those conditions.

One problem is that cigar packages are not required to display health warnings. In addition, cigar manufacturers, importers, and distributors aren't required to submit to the federal government a list of ingredients added to tobacco in the manufacture of cigars. Since there are no health warnings on cigars, some people assume that cigars aren't harmful. Wrong again!

Dentists are often the first to find oral cancers caused by cigarette and cigar smoking.

Many other "myths" surround the cigar craze:

Myth #1: Cigar smoking is a safe alternative to cigarettes.
Fact: Overall cancer death rates among men who smoke cigars are 34 percent higher than cancer death rates among nonsmokers. Cigar smokers have higher death rates from chronic obstructive pulmonary disease, and they're four to ten times more likely to die from laryngeal, oral, and esophageal cancers than nonsmokers. This rate increases when cigar smoking is combined with heavy drinking.

Myth #2: Cigars aren't addictive.
Fact: Cigars as well as cigarettes contain nicotine, an addictive drug, which reaches the brain faster than drugs that enter the body intravenously.

Myth #3: Cigar smoking doesn't cause lung cancer, emphysema, or chronic bronchitis because you don't inhale.
Fact: Even if cigar smokers don't *think* they inhale, they do at least to some extent. The secondhand smoke is in the air all around them. And, holding a lit cigar in the mouth also leads to inhaling smoke.

Similar myths have been used in the past to promote pipe smoking, chewing tobacco and snuff. Who knows what the next "safe" tobacco product will be?

Is Anything "Safe?"

It's actually difficult to identify health advantages for any of the supposedly "safer" tobacco products. In fact, there is no such thing as a "safe" cigarette. Consider filter-tipped cigarettes, for example. Filters reduce the health risks, but nicotine and other chemicals still get through, so the damaging effects are the same.

In addition, as you read earlier, smokers may inhale more often and more deeply with filtered or low-tar brands to get their usual amount of nicotine so they are exposed to an even higher level of carbon monoxide and other toxic substances. That's also a problem with cutting down on smoking rather than quitting entirely. Although light smokers have less chance of developing emphysema and other diseases, they are still inhaling toxic chemicals. So light smokers are by no means safe from smoking-related diseases.

What about menthol cigarettes? Low-tar and menthol cigarettes share the same disadvantages. The advertisements say that menthol prevents throat irritation. But because menthol cigarettes give a feeling of coolness, smokers tend to inhale them more deeply or hold the smoke in for a longer time. As a result, menthol cigarettes may cause more harm to smokers than regular brands.

If It's Legal to Advertise Them, They Must Be Safe. Right?

Few states have restrictions on tobacco advertising and promotion—and these restrictions tend to be mild. Some studies suggest that the lack of tough government restrictions on cigarette marketing leads people to infer that smoking must not be as dangerous as antismoking advocates claim. The industry's huge public relations and advertising budgets strive to reassure smokers. They portray the health effects of smoking as a controversy rather than acknowledging that cigarettes kill.

Cigarette manufacturers spend more money on advertising and marketing than is spent on any other consumer product in the United States. As you know, we are inundated by tobacco ads in newspapers, magazines and billboards. Cigarette companies also spread the word through in-store displays, distribution of free samples, and sales of related goods such as cigarette lighters and T-shirts. They also purchase "name recognition" by sponsoring civic and sporting events and by paying movie producers to give cigarette brands "visibility" in popular films. All of which are examples of their continuing ability to line their pockets at the expense of your health.

> **Health-care professionals urge people to avoid tobacco in all forms—including cigars and chewing tobacco. In 1996 alone, more than 58,000 new cases of oral cancer were diagnosed, and more than 9,000 deaths were recorded.**

Speaking of Money...

Cigarettes cost Americans over *100 billion dollars* annually in tobacco-related health expenses and lost productivity. That's about $398 per American per year. The American

Lung Association estimates that the cost of treating smoking-related disorders, and dealing with the resultant lost productivity, amounts to $3.90 for each pack of cigarettes sold in the U.S. That means that all of us, smokers and nonsmokers alike, are subsidizing smoking at a rate of about $4.00 a pack! And these estimates don't include burns suffered in smoking-related fires, low birth-weight and premature births related to prenatal smoking, or illnesses traceable to secondhand smoke exposure. In fact, total lifetime excess medical-care costs for smokers exceed those for nonsmokers by *$501 billion.*

Of course, at about $2.00 a pack, a pack-a-day smoker spends over $700 a year just for the cigarettes.

Attitudes Are Changing

But there has been a revolution in Americans' attitudes and health behavior. At the time of the first Surgeon General's Report on Smoking in 1964, about half of the adult population smoked. Today, that figure has dropped to about one-quarter of the population. Smoking is banned in many public places and on most airplane flights in the continental United States. Most hospitals and even many restaurants have gone smoke-free.

Public attitudes toward smoking have undergone a tremendous turnaround. Many smokers are recognizing that the nicotine in tobacco is addictive, and they don't like to think of themselves as addicts. They don't want to feel that they're controlled by anything.

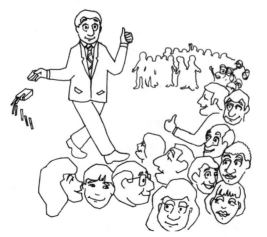

Over 46 million Americans have quit smoking

The largest government survey on smoking ever performed found that a clear majority of smokers as well as nonsmokers agreed that, "Smoking is enough of a health hazard that something should be done about it." Nine out of ten smokers were negative about their own smoking.

In fact, more than 46 million American adults—nearly half of all who ever smoked—have quit smoking.

So What to Do With All of This

This chapter has helped you look at the many ways smoking hurts and kills people, and the reasons more people don't "get it" about smoking. Reading these things in a book or hearing them from your doctor—or even the Surgeon General—won't *make* you quit. But focusing on risks that personally affect you can help you develop the motivation to quit and, most important, stay quit. Because the benefits of quitting far outweigh the advantages of smoking—the damage you have done can be undone with each passing day.

LONG-TERM BENEFITS OF QUITTING

AT 5 YEARS

▶ From five to fifteen years after quitting, stroke risk is reduced to that of people who have never smoked.

AT 10 YEARS

▶ Risk of lung cancer drops to as little as one-half that of continuing smokers.

▶ Risk of cancer of the mouth, throat, esophagus, bladder, kidney, and pancreas decreases.

▶ Risk of ulcer decreases.

AT 15 YEARS

▶ Risk of coronary heart disease is now similar to that of people who have never smoked.

▶ Risk of death returns to nearly the level of people who have never smoked.

You'll need some very convincing reasons to give up your smoking habit. In fact, it will help you in quitting to think about

CONSIDER YOUR REASONS TO QUIT

Finish the following sentence as many times as you can:

If I didn't smoke, I could _____

For example,

If I didn't smoke, I could *stop coughing so much.*

If I didn't smoke, I could *have enough wind to play with my children.*

If I didn't smoke, I could *be less likely to die of lung cancer like my father did.*

Now you try it:

(If you need more room, continue on a separate page)

If I didn't smoke, I could _____

If I didn't smoke, I could _____

If I didn't smoke, I could _____

If I didn't smoke, I could _____

If I didn't smoke, I could _____

If you're running out of ideas, think of your goals this way:

The best thing about quitting smoking is that_____

_____

_____

The second best thing about quitting smoking is that _____

_____

_____

The third best thing about quitting smoking is that_____

_____

_____

why you want to quit—both the risks you'll avoid and the benefits you'll get from quitting. Here's how to make your list.

You probably came up with many more good reasons for not smoking than you thought you would. So what's holding you back? If obstacles still stand in your path, learn how to work around them in the next chapter.

CHAPTER 3

A New Lifestyle: Overcoming Your Obstacles to Quitting

Before you quit smoking, you need three things:

First, you need to make up your mind that you really want to quit.
Second, you need to find the best way to quit—a way that fits with *your* needs, *your* lifestyle, and *your* smoking habit.
Third, you need some *healthy selfishness*.

What Is Healthy Selfishness?

The first two are self-explanatory. But what's healthy selfishness ?

▶   You have the **right** and the **responsibility** to do what's necessary for you to reach your reasonable goal.
▶   You want to quit smoking. This is a reasonable goal. So, you have the right to ask those around you to cooperate with your efforts.

This is healthy selfishness.

Learning how to deal with smoking triggers, how to use self-control, and how to be more skilled in dealing with the feelings you now handle with cigarettes is incredibly difficult. You can't be smoke-free unless you accept the fact that you have a right to change yourself, to do something good for yourself. You must also accept the responsibility of caring for yourself—ultimately, only you put the cigarette in your mouth.

Why don't we do the things we need for ourselves? Sometimes we don't really feel we have the right. We need to recognize that we do, and that it's fair to ask others to cooperate in our efforts to quit smoking.

Let's look at an example of what this means. Marie gets upset after dinner if her kids don't settle down to do their homework. She's tired by this point in the evening, so arguing over homework

> **You have a right to do something good for yourself.**

usually leads her to smoke several cigarettes. She knows this will be a hard time to resist smoking after she quits.

Marie has a right to ask her husband to help her avoid this stress. For example, he might watch the kids on school nights for the first few weeks after Marie quits. He might think it is overly selfish for her to ask this of him. But actually, this is *healthy selfishness*. Her quitting smoking is worth his effort.

Certainly, Marie wants her husband's cooperation. Of course, she needs to be cooperative, too. Marie's husband may suggest that he can't start watching the kids on school nights until next week, when his special project is completed at work. Marie and he can work on cooperating with each other, finding a solution that's agreeable to both of them.

Rights and Responsibilities

Healthy selfishness has two basic components:

1. The *right* to do the things you need, and
2. The *responsibility* to do them.

When you feel comfortable with both components, you feel confident.

Returning to the example of Marie, it is Marie's *right* to seek her husband's help. But if she doesn't ask him to help, she is *responsible* for the consequences. It would be unfair to blame him if she ends up smoking again.

Think about your right and responsibility to do the things you need.

▶ **Do you really feel you have the right to take care of yourself?**
▶ **Do you hesitate to ask others to help you meet your needs?**

Quitting smoking is probably the most important and most difficult thing you'll do all year. Isn't it logical to expect cooperation from those around you? After all, if you had the most important and difficult work assignment of the year, you'd expect

Quitting smoking is probably the most important and most difficult thing you'll do all year.

your spouse and family to take on more of the household chores, to be considerate of your needs, to buy take-out food for dinner rather than insisting that you cook. You'd also cut yourself some slack, permitting other work responsibilities to get placed on the back burner for several weeks. Well, quitting smoking deserves all of these considerations.

What's Holding You Back?

Don't blame yourself because you haven't been able to quit smoking yet. If you've tried to quit before and have always gone back to smoking, that's not a good reason to give up hope. Most successful quitters try a few times before they quit for good, and they learn from their mistakes.

Here are some of the roadblocks that often keep people from quitting. Check off the ones that are holding *you* back, then check out the "Blockbusters" for the roadblocks in *your* path:

❑   **I'll gain too much weight.**

Many people *do* gain weight when they quit, because the body burns calories more slowly as it adjusts to becoming nicotine-free. The average weight gain is in the neighborhood of five to ten pounds. Some people gain much less, some gain more. This weight gain is troublesome for many ex-smokers. It will take healthy eating and exercise to lose those unwanted pounds.

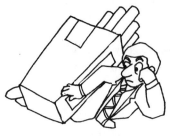

If you slip, try again. And again

Q U I C K   Q U I T   T I P

To help limit weight gain after quitting:

► Eat a well-balanced diet and avoid the excess calories in sugary and fatty foods.

► Satisfy cravings for sweets by eating small pieces of fruit.

► Have low-calorie foods on hand for nibbling.

But rather than becoming discouraged, try to remember an important medical fact you may not have known:

A little extra weight is less risky for you than smoking.

> **Many ex-smokers succeed by stopping, starting, stopping—and then, finally, by quitting and sticking to it.**

Smoking is uniquely dangerous. You'd have to gain eighty or ninety pounds to do as much damage to your health as smoking one pack of cigarettes a day. (See Blockbuster #1 and #2)

❑ My spouse smokes. All my friends smoke. It would be too hard to quit with people smoking around me all the time.

It is harder to stop smoking if the people you spend time with are smoking. Tell your spouse, or your roommate, and your smoking friends that quitting smoking *now* is very important to you. Ask them not to smoke around you and not to offer you cigarettes.

Practice ways to say "no" if someone offers you a cigarette. Ask people to help you, and you'll be surprised how eager they are to watch you for any slip-ups. If you do slip and want to smoke, don't bum a cigarette from anyone else. You must go out and buy your own cigarettes. By the time you do this, the urge may pass. (see Blockbuster #3)

❑ There's too much going on in my life right now.

You probably wouldn't want to plan your quit day right before difficult activities such as moving or changing jobs. And if you're in the midst of a lot of stress, it may be hard to quit.

On the other hand, it may not work to quit when you have nothing but free time. When it comes to giving up cigarettes, that can be just as bad as having too much to do. That's why some people surprise themselves and find it's easier to quit when they're in their regular routine than when they're on vacation. (see Blockbusters #4 and #6)

❑ I wouldn't know what to do without a cigarette.

Do you like the feel of a cigarette in your hand? Do you always reach for a cigarette when you're bored, when you're busy, when you're unhappy, when you're waiting in line, when

> "I told everyone I knew that I had quit smoking. That was really helpful, because people knew that the last thing I needed was the offer of a cigarette." —Lisette, age 19

you're talking on the telephone . . . *whenever!* For you, the real challenge is to find things to do instead of smoking.

For example, if you smoke after dinner, try getting up from the table and taking a brisk walk. If you smoke when you drink, cut down on alcohol or chew on your stirring stick. Be creative! (see Blockbusters #4 and #6)

❏ I'll get too uptight if I stop smoking.

Most smokers say smoking calms them. In fact, when you do quit, at first you will feel more stressed. But there are many better ways to calm down than puffing on a cigarette. One of the best ways is to "Relaxercise," as you'll learn later in this chapter. (see Blockbuster #5)

❏ I don't have the will power to quit.

Yes, you do! Every smoker can quit. Almost 50 percent of smokers—including millions of heavy smokers—have quit. In fact, there are more ex-smokers and nonsmokers than there are smokers in the United States today. **The 7-Steps to a Smoke-Free Life** program will help **you** become an ex-smoker, too.

Making the decision to quit will make it easier for you to stop. So keep reading and you'll have the tools you need to make—and stick with—that decision. (see Blockbuster #6)

> "In the past, I really didn't think it through. I realized that I need to plan what to do in place of smoking. I do have choices."
> —Al, age 64

Blockbusters You Can Count On

You probably spent a number of years creating your smoking pattern. So it's likely that it's going to take a bit of doing to break that pattern. That's why we're supplying some powerful blockbusters to help you break down the roadblocks and obstacles you're likely to encounter.

BLOCKBUSTER #1
A MIRACLE DRUG CALLED EXERCISE

Exercise helps many people quit smoking. It can help you relax. It can give you something to do instead of smoking. It can help you control your weight. It can improve your health. Exercise can be as simple as choosing the stairs instead of the elevator, or getting off the bus a stop or two early and walking the rest of the way. If you want to try a little more, and you're not used to exercise, brisk walking is a good way to start.

> "I found that a lot of my friends have quit smoking, too. And they had some pretty good tips for me."
> —Louis, 27

If you can't walk outside, walk at your local mall. Many shopping centers have "Mallwalkers" programs to encourage exercisers. Often, registered walkers are allowed into the mall before opening time, so they have free space to swing their arms and take big strides. Some programs even offer prizes and special discounts to walkers.

About a half hour of walking at a steady pace three or four times a week is good for your body. Most people can handle that much exercise without too much trouble. Of course, you can also choose other activities, such as running, cycling, swimming, dancing, or gardening.

If you're over 40 or have any physical problems (heart disease, high blood pressure, shortness of breath, joint pain,) check with your doctor first to plan an exercise program that's right for you.

QUICK QUIT TIP
If you cannot walk outside, walk at your local mall.
Before your Quit Day, talk with your physician about
an exercise program that is right for you.

BLOCKBUSTER #2 BATTLING THE BULGES

Many people gain weight after giving up smoking. Stopping smoking slows down your body chemistry as you gradually return to a state of well-being. Also, food tastes better, so you may eat more. You may also find that you're reaching for food instead of cigarettes when you want something to do with your hands.

Smokers weigh less on average than nonsmokers. This and other data indicate that smoking unnaturally alters your metabolism. So, when people quit smoking, they don't suddenly develop a weight problem. Rather, their metabolism goes back to normal and they gain weight, to reach the approximate averages (for sex and height) of the rest of the population.

So if you've been smoking to maintain a slim figure, you have not discovered the one way in which smoking is healthy! The weight you might gain when you quit is much less of a health hazard than your smoking. And the distribution of your pounds— the ratio of your waist to your hips— actually improves with smoking cessation.

Read on for some quick tips on how to cope with your concern about weight gain once you quit.

QUICK QUIT TIP:
When You're Feeling Hungry

▶ Drink a large glass of a low-calorie beverage. You'll feel less hungry.

▶ Keep your hands busy. Try sewing, working on a puzzle, writing a letter, washing your hair.

▶ Learn to live with a little hunger. It may disappear in a short time.

▶ Eat slowly. Don't eat on the run, or you'll end up eating more.

▶ Make a list—like this—of five things you'll do if you're tempted toward eating:

1. Wash your face.
2. Weigh yourself.
3. Stand up and stretch
4. Trim, clean, or file your nails.
5. Make one phone call to a friend

Another tip: Stock up on smart snacks like the ones listed here. It's much healthier to reach for an apple than for a cigarette.

QUICK QUIT TIP:

Smart Snacks

When you want something sweet, try . . .

▶ berries
▶ plums
▶ fresh or canned pineapple

▶ pears
▶ cantaloupe
▶ a frozen fruit bar
▶ peaches

For a crunchy treat, try . . .

▶ apples
▶ fresh vegetables–carrots, celery, broccoli
▶ popcorn (popped without fat)
▶ graham or wheat crackers

For a chewy nibble, try ...

▶ $1/2$ whole wheat or pumpernickel bagel or
a slice of plain raisin bread
▶ raisins
▶ cereal, like shredded or puffed wheat (without milk)
▶ small bran muffin
▶ $1/2$ whole wheat English muffin

BLOCKBUSTER #3 ASSERTIVE RESPONSES

We often smoke when we feel frustrated or when others treat us badly. Nicotine helps reduce that frustration. So how will you manage once you've given up cigarettes?

One way is to practice being assertive. Assertive responses help you keep your self-respect and build self-esteem, so that you'll be more likely to listen to yourself when it comes to resisting an urge to smoke.

Assertive responses are positive, direct, yet controlled responses you can use to deal with aggravating situations. Such responses let you express your feelings, rather than attacking others or losing control. By being assertive, you stay focused on your own needs and perceptions. In contrast, with aggression, you become focused on changing the other person.

Here's an example. You've been waiting in a very long line at the bank when a young man walks in, sees a friend on the line, and edges into the line in front of his friend, a few places ahead of you.

An *aggressive response* to this situation would be to shout, "Who do you think you are? You can't cut in. Wait your turn like the rest of us!" Even if this does express your feelings, you've lost control, and that loss of control doesn't do your self-respect much good. You probably feel pretty tense as a result, which means an urge for a smoke.

A *passive response* would be to do absolutely nothing or to mutter to yourself. Like the aggressive response, it makes you feel out of control. You've lost a lot of self-respect and you've completely suppressed your feelings. Again, your tension has increased, and you feel like smoking.

An *assertive response* provides a calm, yet controlled, way of expressing your feelings. You might say, in a normal tone of voice: "Excuse me. I see that you're in a hurry, but I'm in a hurry, too. All of us have been waiting on this line for quite a while. I'd appreciate it if you would wait for your turn, too." Even if the person continues to be unreasonable, you've maintained your self-respect and haven't caused yourself additional anxiety.

Just as you *learned* to smoke cigarettes, you can *learn* to be more assertive. Approach each situation directly. Use a neutral tone of voice. Express your feelings openly and honestly, without losing control of them. It takes some practice (so did learning to smoke!), but once you master it, you'll have more control over every area of your life.

PRACTICE ASSERTIVE RESPONSES

You know the old saying "Practice makes perfect," so try some practice in making assertive responses. Your response should express your feelings without losing control of them. Keep in mind how assertive responses can help you in your efforts to become a non-smoker.

Situation: You are at a party and are trying not to smoke. A friend who knows you're trying to quit comes up and offers you a cigarette.
What is your assertive response? _____

_____

Situation: You and your partner go out for dinner and request a seat in the non-smoking section of the restaurant. Midway through dinner, a man seated at the table next to you lights up a cigarette.
What is your assertive response? _____

_____

BLOCKBUSTER #4 CREATIVE ALTERNATIVES

Does getting angry always make you want to light up? Do you smoke more when you're frustrated by problems you can't solve or situations you can't seem to manage? Does feeling bored, or sitting around doing nothing, increase your smoking, too? Do you also smoke if there's not too much going on and you can't do anything about it?

Well, you can do something about all of these things. You have to think of some creative alternatives.

Consider this: What would you do if someone put you in a locked room with no cigarettes and told you you'd have to stay there for a full hour before the lock would automatically open? Close your eyes and picture yourself in the room.

Did you picture yourself sitting in a chair in a totally bare place, with absolutely nothing to do? That *would* be hard to manage without smoking, even for an hour.

But now imagine that the room is filled to the brim with pencils, pens, books, games, crafts items, exercise equipment, foods, a television, a radio, a stereo, a telephone, even a computer. With all that stuff around to keep you busy, it wouldn't be quite so hard to manage an hour without cigarettes, would it?

Well, most of that stuff is probably in your very own house. And you can use all of it when you're trying not to smoke. You just have to remember that it's there and use it creatively. For example, here are some things that have worked for other smokers:

QUICK QUIT TIP

Creative Alternatives to Smoking

If you're bored and trying not to smoke:

- Hold a fake cigarette.
- Take a walk.
- Doodle.
- Chew gum.
- Call a friend.
- See a movie.
- Give yourself a manicure/pedicure.
- Give your partner a massage
- Do a puzzle.
- Exercise.
- Crochet.
- Work on a hobby.
- Eat a low-calorie snack.
- Make a list of list of things to do.
- Read a newspaper.

If you're stressed or unhappy and trying not to smoke:

▶ Squeeze a ball.
▶ Hit a pillow.
▶ Yell and scream.
▶ Do aerobics.
▶ Jump rope.
▶ Play with your child or pet.

▶ Practice deep breathing.
▶ Weed your garden.
▶ Throw darts.
▶ Crush paper.
▶ Build something.

BLOCKBUSTER #5 "RELAXERCISE" TO STAY CALM

Deep breathing is a very effective way of coping with the tension you may experience from giving up and staying off cigarettes. Here's a simple deep-breathing exercise you can do while sitting or standing, whenever you're feeling the need to calm down. When you "Relaxercise," you'll feel relaxed, without smoking.

Here's how to do it:

RELAXERCISE TO STAY CALM

▶ Think about something that makes you feel good.
▶ Relax your shoulders.
▶ Close your mouth and inhale through your nose as slowly and deeply as you can.
▶ Hold your breath while you count to four, keeping your shoulders relaxed.
▶ Exhale slowly, letting out all of the air from your lungs, as if you were blowing out a candle.
▶ Repeat this inhale-exhale cycle five times.

Relaxercise at least once a day from now on. Try it more often once you stop smoking.

> "At first, I thought the Relaxercise was silly. And it felt strange. But after a while it was natural. It works! Do it when you feel an urge to smoke. It will make you feel better."
> —James, age 48

BLOCKBUSTER #6 DO POWER— NOT WILL POWER— AND CREATIVE PROBLEM SOLVING

Many smokers—especially smokers who have tried to quit before and failed—think they just don't have the will power to stop smoking. A lot of people think that will power is either something you have or don't have. And, if you're still smoking, you may think you don't have it—or at least not when it comes to quitting smoking.

It turns out that people who we think have "will power" aren't just willing or wishing for things—they *do things* to get what they want. So for the time being, forget about *will* power. Instead, concentrate on things you can do—boost your **"Do Power."**

What's **Do Power**? It's any creative strategy that keeps temptations from getting in the way of your goals and helps you stay in control. For example, one clever man who was trying to quit smoking noticed that when he drank coffee, he strongly desired a cigarette. By switching to tea for a month, he managed not to smoke at meals or on breaks from work.

There are three critical ingredients in **Do Power:**

1. Anticipate temptations before they occur.

2. Use Creative Problem Solving. Figure out specific ways to change or avoid situations that may tempt you or cause you to relapse. Try to make them life-enhancing so that you don't feel deprived.

3. Do something. Waiting for the devil to get behind you won't work. You need to carry out the plan before the temptation is staring you in the face.

Of the three, Creative Problem Solving is the key ingredient in **Do Power**. What clever strategies can you think of to manage situations that trigger your smoking?

Here are some examples:

Temptation	Creative Problem Solving
Friends who offer me cigarettes when we go drinking together:	▶ Stay away from the bars the first 3–4 weeks after you quit. ▶ Ask your friends to do something else with you instead of drinking so you won't be tempted.
Coffee break at work:	▶ Tell everybody you've quit and ask them not to offer you a cigarette. ▶ Go for a 10-minute walk instead of a coffee break. ▶ Go someplace nearby that makes gourmet coffee, something better than the swill in the break room!

Spouse smokes after dinner:
- ▶ Ask your spouse not to smoke in the house after dinner for the first 2–3 weeks after you quit.
- ▶ Go for a walk by yourself after dinner.

"Quitting is easy. It's staying off that's the hard part. It really isn't a question of will power. There are certain skills you can learn that can help you to quit. If you practice and persevere, you can do it. I know—I did it!"
—Harold, age 58

Warning about Creative Problem Solving Strategies: A great strategy for one person may sound silly or unrealistic to another. A friend controlled the tendency to nibble before dinner by wearing a surgical mask while preparing the meal! Sounds a bit unusual, but it worked — for her. What you need to do is think about what your *specific* temptations are and then identify Creative Problem Solving strategies that *make sense* for you. Use the above examples to get you started, but don't be discouraged if they sound strange to you.

The Odds Are with You

The key to staying off cigarettes is to prepare yourself in advance. You have to rehearse what you will do when you get the urge to smoke. Now you have a whole barrage of Blockbusters to help you along the way.

You may still be worrying, "Can I really do it? Can I really stop smoking?" *Absolutely!* Statistics indicate that you're indeed very likely to succeed. Here are the figures:

▶ More than 46 million American adults—nearly half of those who have ever smoked—have quit smoking.

▶ About 70 percent of ex-smokers had to make one or two attempts to quit before they finally succeeded. And most of the rest relapsed one more time before they stayed quit. So, no matter how many times you've tried and failed, you can do it!

▶ Each year about *1.3 million smokers* quit successfully.

As you can see, the odds are definitely with you. So turn to the next chapter now and learn about the seven important steps that will finally make *you* an ex-smoker.

PART TWO

7 Steps to Quitting Smoking

CHAPTER 4

7 Important Steps

As you begin the **7 Steps to a Smoke-Free Life** program, it may help you to know about the experts who have developed the foundation of this successful plan. For over twenty years, the American Lung Association has recruited teams of physicians, psychologists, and health educators to research the very best way to help people stop smoking. And they have tested their strategies on thousands of smokers in cities all around the United States. The American Lung Association's behavior change approach to smoking cessation has worked for thousands of smokers. **7 Steps to a Smoke-Free Life** will work for you, too.

As the name indicates, the program has seven integral parts, namely:

THE 7-STEP "START OF A SMOKE-FREE LIFE" PLAN

Step 1: Understand Your Habit and Addiction
  ▶ Why do you smoke?
  ▶ How to identify your smoking triggers.

Step 2: Build Your Motivation to Quit
  ▶ How to gain the resolve to change your behavior.
  ▶ Identifying your personal reasons for quitting.

Step 3: Develop Your Quitting Plan
  ▶ How to personalize a quit program that suits your needs.
  ▶ Are nicotine replacement therapies right for you?

Step 4: Prepare for Your Quit Day
- How to break up habits.
- Dealing with temptations.
- Getting the cooperation you need.

Step 5: Quit
- What a new nonsmoker should anticipate.
- How to successfully manage the first 24 hours.
- You planned your work—now work your plan.

Step 6: Fighting Temptations—The First Two Weeks
- How to stick with your plan.
- Emergency treatment to recover from a relapse.
- Fight your inner culprit.

Step 7: Staying Focused—The First Six Months
- The difference between urges and thoughts.
- Using your new coping skills.
- How to deal with weight gain.
- How you can reward your achievement.

The **7 Steps to a Smoke-Free Life** program will first help you to understand your individual smoking habit. Next, it will help you increase and develop the personal motivation to quit. You then will develop an individualized plan for quitting. And finally, you will learn maintenance skills to help you stay off cigarettes. No single quit-smoking method works for everyone. So the program incorporates many well-known techniques, tools, and tips that have been tested for several decades. The more techniques you use, the more likely you will stay quit.

Set Your Own Timetable

The **7 Steps to a Smoke-Free Life** is a simple program, but it's not simple-minded. There's a lot of flexibility built in, so you won't have to gauge your progress against an inflexible calendar in which a single day's misstep can trip you up. Instead, you'll develop your own timetable for quitting, based on your lifestyle and your personal needs.

The program is especially useful for people who have tried to quit before and failed. You can use your past experiences as positive examples of what worked best for you

> **Work *with* the program and it will work for *you*.**

and what didn't. **7 Steps** will help you gain more insight into the psychological needs that fuel your craving for cigarettes. You'll learn how to adjust to a smoke-free life, and how to work through temptations and cravings. You'll also know what to do if a setback occurs and how to get back in the smoke-free groove. This time, you'll quit for good!

CHAPTER 5

Step 1
Understand Your Habit and Your Addiction

Almost every smoker has two basic reasons for continuing to smoke:

1. The nicotine in cigarettes is addictive, and
2. Smoking provides a sense of pleasure. It improves your mood, improves alertness, increases your energy, and relieves stress.

These pleasures are completely normal. But unfortunately, this method of achieving pleasure has a high price: illness or even death. Quitting something pleasurable is never easy. The good news is that you can quit smoking if you have sufficient motivation, an understanding of your addiction, the strength to accept a personal challenge, and—most important—an effective quit smoking plan.

Why Do You Smoke?

Simply learning about the effects that cigarettes have on the body isn't enough to help most people stop smoking. What's more important is to pinpoint the core of your smoking problem: nicotine addiction. That's the crucial beginning of this quit-smoking program.

But that's not all. You must also recognize the psychological reasons you smoke. For example, every smoker had different psychological motives for beginning to smoke in the first place; peer pressure, stress, and curiosity are some of the common reasons. Smokers also have different reasons for wanting to free themselves from their addiction; health concerns, appearance concerns, family pressure, workplace restrictions, and money are common reasons.

The underlying premise of **7 Steps to a Smoke-Free Life** is that smoking is *a learned habit driven by a powerful addictive drug—nicotine.*

Smoking is not a natural act. You had to learn how to smoke. When you first tried cigarettes, they probably made you feel sick. It may have taken awhile, but you overcame that sick feeling. You had a strong desire to practice and to learn. You conditioned your body to accept the assault of the chemicals in cigarette smoke.

Smoking is a complex habit because people learn to smoke to fill so many needs. For many people, their initial need was acceptance by their peers, or a desire to feel "grown up." You may have also found that smoking was a good way to relieve tiredness, reduce stress, control hunger, and increase your social enjoyment.

So, you repeated the act of smoking again and again, until smoking became associated with a broad range of positive effects. Now, smoking has become linked with many rewards in many circumstances.

How to Unlearn an Automatic Behavior

In psychological terms you acquired the learned habit of smoking—you were conditioned to smoke in response to a broad range of environmental stimuli. The **7 Steps to a Smoke-Free Life** program is a step-by-step behavior change approach that will help you *unlearn* the automatic behavior of smoking.

It's helpful to distinguish between *habit* and *addiction.* A **habit** is a well learned behavior. An **addiction** is a highly repetitive or compulsive pattern of using a drug. Numerous research studies have shown that nicotine is the drug in tobacco that causes addiction.

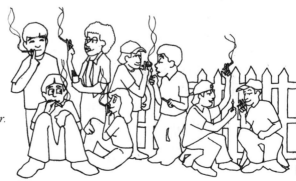

You LEARNED to be a smoker. Now you can LEARN to be a nonsmoker.

The addictive process and the conditioning process by which smoking becomes a habit work together to making smoking a lethal behavior that is very resistant to change. As discussed in Chapter 1, the conditioning makes the addiction worse and the addiction makes the conditioning worse. The key is to combat both processes together.

What Are Your Triggers?

As you have seen, there are many different reasons why you smoke—habit, addiction, social enjoyment, stress relief, hunger control, advertising messages, and more. In fact, your reasons often change from day to day. One day you may smoke a lot because you're feeling stressed. Another day, you may be at a gathering with friends where you all smoke together. On other days, you may be home alone with nothing to do, so you smoke to reduce your feelings of boredom.

Smoking also fills different needs at different times of the day. Smoking may give you something to do with your hands when you're on the phone or waiting on line. Having a cigarette may help you slow down and take a break when you need to relax.

Each time you smoke you reinforce the connection between the act of smoking and your current activity or situation. You no longer think about needing something to do with your hands. Instead, you automatically smoke whenever you're on the telephone, or when you're waiting on line, or when you're taking a coffee break.

These feelings and situations serve as **triggers**—that is, cues to light up. Think of yourself for a moment. What are some of the triggers you have had today? What situations caused you to have a cigarette?

Some activities are so strongly connected to smoking that you can't imagine doing them without a cigarette. For instance, do you always smoke while driving in your car? At the end of a meal? When talking on the telephone?

Smoking is such an automatic behavior that most people don't think about what triggers it, or how important any particular trigger is. You don't think about the cigarettes you smoke, you just smoke them. It's like being on automatic pilot. Sometimes, people even light up a cigarette and then realize they already have one lit in the ashtray.

If you try to break the smoking habit by just throwing your cigarettes away, the triggers can be overwhelming. In Step 4, you'll learn how to break up the triggers *before* you quit, and make plans to cope with any remaining triggers *after* you quit, rather than throwing your cigarettes away and praying.

How to Play "Pack Track"

Right now, you may be thinking, "I smoke because I like it! That's what really counts." Well, of course. But there are probably many reasons that go into your liking to smoke. The goal is to pinpoint the major reasons you have for smoking. If you know where, when, and why you light up, you can plan ahead for those times and those reasons.

To get started, try playing **Pack Track**. You may have tried this already, while reading Chapter 1. If so, skip past the next paragraph.

If you're playing Pack Track for the first time, photocopy page 59 of this book and cut out a Pack Track card. You'll notice that each card is about the size of your cigarette pack. Use one Pack Track card for each pack of cigarettes you smoke over the next few days. You can either attach the card to the pack with a rubber band or put it inside the cellophane. That way, it will be with you all the time and you can play Pack Track every time you smoke.

Every time you smoke, write down the time, the mood you're in, and how much you need that cigarette. If you really want to learn a lot, keep track of where you are when you smoke each cigarette.

- ▶ If you're in a **good** mood, put a check mark under the smiling face.
- ▶ If you're in a **bad** mood, check the sad face.
- ▶ If you feel **in-between**, check the middle face.
- ▶ If you **really want** that cigarette, check "YES" (capital letters)
- ▶ If you want it but **not a lot**, check "yes" (small letters)
- ▶ If it's **no big deal**, check "???"

Playing this game for at least three to five days is best. Try to include both weekends and weekdays. Then look over your cards and see what patterns you have set up. Many smokers check a lot of boxes in all categories.

First Look At Your Faces:

▶ If you checked a lot of **happy, smiling faces**, then a lot of your cigarettes come when you're feeling relaxed.

▶ If you checked a lot of the **"in-between" blah faces**, it's likely that you smoke many of your cigarettes when you're bored.

▶ If you checked a lot of **unhappy, sad faces**, it's likely that you smoke many of your cigarettes as a way to control your mood. Many people who are having a rough time dealing with work problems, divorce, societal prejudices, depression, and other psychological problems take up smoking as an antidote. See the box on Depression, Feeling Sad, and Smoking, below.

DEPRESSION, FEELING SAD, AND SMOKING

Most of us have periods of "blue" moods or anxiety, and most smokers smoke to control these moods—remember nicotine helps lift our mood and contain anxiety. So most smokers will have to develop some alternative ways of coping with sadness and anxiety after they quit.

For some smokers, depression really makes quitting very difficult. If you think this might be a problem for you, you might want to ask your doctor for some advice or seek help yourself from a psychologist or other therapist or counselor.

If you are seeing a psychologist or other counselor for depression or anxiety, tell your therapist about your desire to quit smoking and ask them to help you figure out better ways to cope with low mood when you quit.

A new development that may be of help is the use of antidepressant medication to assist in quitting—this is covered in Step 3.

Think about how much you needed each cigarette:

▶ *If you checked mostly* "**YES**," you may be especially addicted to nicotine. As you'll learn later, nicotine replacement products may be especially helpful to you during the early weeks of quitting.

▶ *If you checked mostly* "**yes**" *or* "**???**," you are probably smoking in association with situations that occur each day, such as waking up, eating meals, talking on the telephone, and watching television.

Now, think about the time and place you smoked each cigarette:

▶ *Where were you* when you had the highest number of cigarettes?

▶ *What times of day* were you most likely to light up?

▶ What were you doing or feeling?

Pack Tracks

DATE:

No.	Time	Need ???	Need yes	Need YES	Mood 😃	Mood 😐	Mood 😧
1							
2							
3							
4							
5							
6							
7							
8							
9							
10							

© AMERICAN LUNG ASSOCIATION, 1993

DATE:

No.	Time	Need ???	Need yes	Need YES	Mood 😃	Mood 😐	Mood 😧
1							
2							
3							
4							
5							
6							
7							
8							
9							
10							

© AMERICAN LUNG ASSOCIATION, 1993

Fold

DATE:

No.	Time	Need ???	Need yes	Need YES	Mood 😃	Mood 😐	Mood 😧
1							
2							
3							
4							
5							
6							
7							
8							
9							
10							

© AMERICAN LUNG ASSOCIATION, 1993

DATE:

No.	Time	Need ???	Need yes	Need YES	Mood 😃	Mood 😐	Mood 😧
1							
2							
3							
4							
5							
6							
7							
8							
9							
10							

© AMERICAN LUNG ASSOCIATION, 1993

Cut

These places, times, and feelings may be triggers that cause you to smoke. In Step 4, you'll use this information to plan things to do instead of smoking.

What did you learn about your smoking habit? Do you smoke more than you thought, or less? What was the mood that showed up most often on your cards? How many times was your need very high? This information is going to be used extensively in Step 4 of the program, as you prepare for your Quit Day. It will help you figure out how to break up your habit both before and after you quit smoking.

Dealing with Your Addiction

The **7 Steps to a Smoke-Free Life** program works for all types of smokers. It doesn't matter if you smoke when you're happy or unhappy, or if you smoke at certain times of day. It also doesn't matter that you're addicted to cigarettes.

The 1988 Surgeon General's Report concluded that cigarettes and other forms of tobacco *are* addicting. The fact that nicotine ingestion controls when and how much people smoke defies the myth that cigarette smoking is a casual habit, governed only by the desire or whim of the smoker. In fact, the 1988 Report, completed under C. Everett Koop, noted that cigarette smoking is as addictive as heroin or cocaine.

Many smokers think that if they're addicted they won't be able to quit and so there's no use trying. "Addiction" does not mean "can't be changed." The fact is that addictions can be broken. Quitting smoking is difficult, but thousands of smokers have done it. *You can do it, too.*

Do you think you are addicted to cigarettes? To find out, ask yourself the five questions on page 61.

Many smokers answer "yes" to two or more questions. If you did, that's an indication that addiction to nicotine is a powerful trigger in your smoking habit. You're likely to notice physical symptoms when you stop smoking and nicotine is withdrawn from your system. These symptoms may last a few days. But the good news is that, addictive as it may be, nicotine leaves your body quite quickly, as soon as you stop smoking.

ADDICTION QUIZ

Circle YES or NO

▶ Do you smoke your first cigarettes within 30 minutes of waking up in the morning?

YES   NO

▶ Do you smoke 20 cigarettes (one pack) or more each day?

YES   NO

▶ At times when you can't smoke or don't have any cigarettes, do you feel a craving for one?

YES   NO

▶ Is it tough to keep from smoking for more than a few hours?

YES   NO

▶ When you are sick enough to stay in bed, do you still smoke?

YES   NO

Some people mistakenly believe that cutting down on smoking, changing their cigarette smoking patterns, or switching to brands that are advertised as "low tar" or "low nicotine" will be enough to help them overcome their nicotine addiction. But these strategies are, at best, only minimally effective, since smokers almost always compensate by increasing the number of puffs they take with each cigarette, or by puffing more deeply, so any "health" benefits are lost.

Of course, the cravings will continue longer than a few days, but there are many ways to deal with them. Some addicted smokers are helped by "nicotine fading," a strategy of switching to cigarettes with lower amounts of nicotine and gradually smoking less, as you prepare to quit totally. Other addicted smokers may want to use a temporary nicotine substitute, such as nicotine gum or the nicotine patch. We'll discuss these methods in Step 3.

CHAPTER 6

Step 2
Build Your Motivation to Quit

Wouldn't it be wonderful if you could just wake up one morning and not want to smoke? Unfortunately, wanting to quit just isn't enough.

If you're reading this book, you do want to quit, and you're not alone. Three out of four smokers would like to quit. Five out of six say they would not start smoking in the first place if they had the choice to make over again. In fact, most smokers eventually do quit smoking. The 1989 Surgeon General's Report estimated that almost 50 percent of all adults who had ever smoked regularly had quit.

But quitting smoking isn't easy. You've probably gone to bed at night saying, "Okay, this is my last cigarette." Then you woke up the next morning and couldn't keep from lighting up. Studies have shown that many successful quitters failed in their first attempts to quit. There's actually little connection between the number of previous quit attempts and eventual success. So previous failures don't mean that you can't succeed.

Quitting smoking is hard to do. It requires strong motivation. Motivations don't just pop up in your brain. You can take an active part in developing your motivations and making them more effective. That's what Step 2 is all about—building the motivation you need to quit.

Act As If You Can Quit

To start off, think about how you *think* about quitting. Do you think of it as giving something up? Instead, try thinking of it as a positive act—improving your health, taking control of your life—whatever "grabs" you.

It will help you to believe it is *possible* for you to quit. If you have quit before, try reframing your past "failure" as a success. First, you *were* able to quit for some length of time—probably for longer than you thought you could. You learned some things that will help you *this* time. You probably learned you can't "have just one." And maybe you recognized some triggers or temptations you really need to watch out for.

As we pointed out in Chapter 1, there are lots of very understandable reasons why you want to smoke. Also, it's hard for people to make changes. As clear as it may be to you that you need to make a change, change is scary—particularly when it requires changing something as fundamental in your life as smoking has become.

Your Health Concerns

Has your doctor ever told you to give up cigarettes? Studies show that many doctors do advise smokers to quit, but in a way that's easy to ignore. "You really should stop smoking" isn't enough. At that point, most smokers can honestly reply, "Yes, I know I should. And I've tried!"

If your doctor hasn't talked to you about quitting, you may wonder whether it's really so important. It is! And doctors know it's important, but many are frustrated that their patients continue to smoke. Often there is too little time to have long discussions with their patients about things like smoking. Some doctors may think that the importance of quitting smoking "goes without saying." And sometimes smoking may not be discussed when other problems need to be corrected. Whatever your doc-

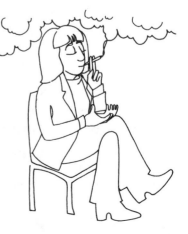

You've had plenty of practice being a smoker. Puff after puff.

tor's motivation, quitting is vitally important to your health. If you have any doubt, just ask your doctor.

We mentioned earlier that, in addition to lung cancer, many people don't realize how often smoking kills people from other cancers, heart disease, and stroke. Many don't realize that smoking multiplies the risks of heart disease, diabetes, and other conditions, making the combination especially lethal.

And fear can be part of the problem. Often smokers deny smoking's health risks because they fear having to quit. They want to "hang on" to what is comfortable. They may also fear that if they acknowledge how harmful smoking is, they come too close to realizing how it may have already harmed them.

How about *you?* How's your health? Do you have some nagging health concerns that you've tried to brush off, out of fear that it really could be something serious? For example, many smokers have a chronic heavy cough, which often brings up mucus. Coughing is an early warning sign of potential lung damage. More severe problems such as shortness of breath, wheezing, and coughing up blood could be a sign of chronic obstructive pulmonary disease, or even lung cancer. Chest pain could be a sign of cardiovascular disease. These are serious problems that should not be ignored.

What are your other health concerns? Think about how these problems might be made worse by your smoking. (Chapter 2 may be worth reviewing here.) It's not pleasant, but if you can recognize your own worries about smoking, it may help motivate you to quit and stay quit.

Social Pressures

Once you've faced your health concerns, you may become more aware of other reasons to stop smoking. For instance, does it seem as if more and more people are asking you not to smoke lately? If so, you're right! The antismoking message is spreading rapidly.

It's a bit ironic that most people start smoking because of social pressures—to fit in with the crowd, to look older, more sophisticated, sexier. Once they become smokers in today's world, however, they're increasingly pressured *not* to smoke.

With this changing social climate, nonsmokers have become braver and bolder about approaching total strangers and demanding, "Your smoke is really bothering me. Would you please put out your cigarette or move to another area."

For some people, this type of pressure can be a motivation to *keep* smoking: "You can't tell me what to do." Ask yourself what *you* most want. If it's to do the many things you enjoy for as long as you can . . . Well, you can figure this one out!

Studies show that the changing norms regarding smoking behavior are also helping people to quit and stay quit. For example, long-term abstinence is more likely if few or none of your friends smoke. Abstinence is also greatly improved with the support and encouragement of nonsmoking friends and relatives.

Nonsmoking at Work

One place where important social norms can encourage non-smoking is at work. Indeed, many workplaces now sponsor smoking cessation clinics. Companies have actually found that they are cost-effective because nonsmokers miss fewer days of work and make less use of their medical benefits. So, quitting smoking will probably help you feel part of the team at work, too.

Even more ambitious than worksite activities, some entire communities are sponsoring smoking cessation campaigns, often accompanied by televised programs

Environmental tobacco smoke causes an estimated 3,000 lung cancer deaths per year in adult nonsmokers.

and distribution of printed materials to every resident. Local schools in many areas of the country also run schoolwide smoking prevention programs, directed at students, and their friends and relatives. For example, many schools participate in the American Lung Association's "Smoke-Free Class of 2000" program. Our country is changing to make nonsmoking the norm—eventually you'll want to be part of this healthy trend rather than "behind the curve."

Personal Concerns

Despite all the antismoking campaigns, health warnings, and educational efforts, most people who stop do so for very personal reasons. Your own reasons for wanting to quit may be very different from someone else's reasons. For example:

▶ An aunt, an uncle, an old friend, or someone you were very fond of may have died from lung cancer, heart disease, or another smoking-related illness. That person can be your inspiration to quit for good.

▶ You're expecting a new baby. If you're pregnant, you know that quitting can protect your unborn child's health. If you're the partner of a pregnant woman, you know that secondhand smoke can be damaging to her health and the baby you will love.

▶ You're getting older and you've become more concerned about your appearance. You're distressed that cigarettes have discolored your teeth and your fingers. Your breath smells bad, too. And you've even learned that smoking causes wrinkles.

> **"I'd feel better and I'd have more energy if I didn't cough so much."**
> **—Rosalind, age 40**

Knowing your own reasons for quitting—and remembering them when times get tough—will be a big help to you in becoming a nonsmoker.

So take the time right now to think of all your personal reasons for wanting to quit. Here's how to do it:

IMPORTANT REASONS I WANT TO QUIT SMOKING

1. **Check the boxes next to the reasons for quitting**
   Go through this list and, using the boxes, check those reasons that are important to you. Give 2 checks to reasons that are especially important to you.
   ❑ I will have more control of my life.
   ❑ I will be healthier.
   ❑ My heart rate and blood pressure will be lower.
   ❑ I'll save lots of money.
   ❑ I'm tired of smoky-smelling breath and clothes.
   ❑ I'll set a better example for my children.
   ❑ I'll have more energy.
   ❑ The chances of fire in my home will decrease.
   ❑ I'll lessen my chances of death from heart disease, chronic bronchitis, emphysema, and cancer.
   ❑ Add more reasons you can think of.
   _____
   _____

2. **Rank your reasons** for quitting in order of importance.
   Put a 1 on the line beside your number one reason for quitting,
   a 2 beside your second most important reason, and so on, until
   you have given a number to all of your reasons for quitting.
3. **List any reasons you can think of for NOT quitting.**
   Put a 1 on the line beside your number one reason for not quit
   ting, a 2 beside your second most important reason, and so on.

Once you have made your list, study it for two minutes a day,
every day. Keep adding to it as new reasons occur to you. Make this
an active process, not just a crumpled list lost in a drawer.

To keep up your resolve, use the card below to record your
own **"Top 5 Reasons to Stop Smoking."** We've included space
on this to note additional reasons so you can update your list as
you progress in your quit smoking program.

MY TOP 5 IMPORTANT REASONS TO STOP SMOKING

1. _____ ___
2. _____ ___
3. _____ ___
4. _____ ___
5. _____ ___

   The Urge Will Pass— Whether You Smoke or Not

*Additional Notes*_____

_____

Your list of **Important Reasons I Want to Quit Smoking**
and your **Top 5 Important Reasons to Stop Smoking** card
will be helpful tools to overcome urges to smoke. Here are three
ways to use them:

1. Keep them close. Make copies of your list and post them in
places you pass frequently (for example, on your refrigerator or at
your workstation).
2. Keep them current. Continue to collect reasons to quit. When

you have an urge to smoke, ask someone for a reason to quit. Every time you hear one you like, add it to your list.

3. Keep the Top 5 Important Reasons to Stop Smoking card convenient. Carry it where you carry your cigarettes. Then when you have an urge to smoke, think about what's important to you.

4. After you quit, continue to carry your **Top 5 Important Reasons.** Pay attention to that quote on the card: "The urge will pass, whether you smoke or not!"

Embrace Your Ambivalence

People are usually a bit nervous when they reach this point in the program. First, because you've played the **Pack Track** game, which tends to make you a lot more aware of how much your cigarettes mean to you And next, because you've zeroed in on the most important personal reasons why you really do want to quit.

Look back at your "Important Reasons I Want to Quit Smoking" questionnaire again. You'll notice that item 4 lists your reasons for *NOT* wanting to quit. That's the crux of the problem: You want to quit, but you also want to keep smoking!

You're probably thinking, "On the one hand, I want to quit because . . . Yet, on the other hand, I really like smoking." It's important to continue this "On the one hand . . . on the other hand" conversation to help you face the issues you are concerned about.

Why? Because it is only by embracing and working with this ambivalence that it can be resolved. Your reasons to be hesitant about quitting are real. Remember the disussion in Chapter 1 of all the reasons there are for smoking? Don't run away from these. Be open to thinking about both these and your reasons for quitting. Then, when you decide you really *do* want to quit, your resolve will be stronger. You will have acknowledged that you do have valid reasons for wanting to keep smoking—it's just that your reasons for wanting to stop are even stronger. You will have made an informed decision.

So, weigh your reasons for smoking and for quitting carefully. Use paper and pencil and write down the reasons why you would make either choice. Then compare them. That way you can make a clear choice between them. When people lose sight of their choices, they begin to feel deprived. And that's when negative thinking takes over. It's important for you to see that there *are* two choices.

But changing a behavior like smoking is as much emotional as it is rational. Smoking has nothing to do with how smart you are. You must bring together what you know in your head and your heart with what you feel in your gut! Then you will begin to increase your desire to quit and your confidence in your ability to do it.

Close Your "Back Doors"

The fear of quitting—of really *never* having another cigarette—makes some people leave open a "back door" as an excuse for going back to smoking. Examples would be: "I'll quit smoking as long as I don't gain more than ten pounds," or "I'll stop smoking as long as I don't have to deal with any big crises." In addition to weight and crises, other back doors are:

- crabbiness
- a minor relapse—"I've failed , so I might as well stop punishing myself."
- family quarrels
- work pressure

Before you quit smoking, you have to close your "back doors." Begin by deciding what you are going to do about each barrier and each roadblock that's holding you back. Review each of the Blockbusters in Chapter 3, so you can say, "I'm going to stop smoking while I practice other stress management techniques," or "I'm going to stop smoking because I've learned other things I can do with my hands instead of smoking," or "I'm going to stop smoking by being more assertive."

Develop Your Self-Confidence

You need two types of confidence to succeed in quitting.

1. **Confidence in the program. 7 Steps to a Smoke-Free Life** works for all kinds of smokers and it will work for you whether you smoke a few cigarettes aday or three packs a day. It has been successful for people who have smoked for fifty years or for just one year.

2. **Confidence in yourself.** You can begin building that confidence by using a positive attitude and **Positive Self-Talk**. For starters, practice saying out loud, "I *can* quit smoking!"

As you go along, make up other **confidence statements** to address your personal concerns. Say, for example, "I can stop smoking *and* maintain my current weight," or "I can stop smoking *and* learn new ways to manage stress," or "I love myself too much to let myself smoke."

Words alone won't be sufficient, though. It also helps to review other things you've done that required priority setting and resisting temptation. Did you learn how to get your taxes done early? Have you lost twenty pounds and kept them off? Have you developed better ways of handling disagreements with your spouse or with your children? Have you struggled to reduce salt or fat in your diet or reduce your daily consumption of coffee? Try to identify what kind of problem-solving you are especially good at, then plan how you can emphasize these strengths and apply them to your quit-smoking efforts.

For example, if you work in an office, have you had trouble dealing with pressure or challenges on the job? Perhaps you found that delegating minor tasks to a junior assistant relieved some of those pressures. Is there some way that delegating some of your work in the office, or at home, will lessen the stress in your life and make quitting smoking easier to manage?

What if you're basically a shy person. Have you been able to call on one or two close friends who introduced you to others and helped you get out more? These same friends may be happy to encourage you during the difficult early days of your quit-smoking program.

As we discussed earlier, you have the right to expect assistance and cooperation in your efforts. In the next chapter—Step 3—you'll learn about other forms of assistance, such as nicotine fading, nicotine replacement therapy, drug treatments, and group support programs.

CHAPTER 7

Step 3
Develop Your Quitting Plan

There are three basic questions you have to answer in developing your personal plan for quitting smoking:

1. What type of program is best for you?
- ❏ A **self-help plan**—If this is your choice, all you need is in this book.
- ❏ A **group support program** or **individual counseling** to supplement the information in this **7 Steps to a Smoke-Free Life** program.

2. What mode of quitting is best for you?
- ❏ **"Cold turkey"**—You set a quit date and, when that day comes, you stop smoking entirely.
- ❏ **Nicotine fading**—a process of changing the type of cigarettes you smoke to gradually reduce your nicotine intake before you quit altogether.

3. Do you want to use medications to boost your efforts?
Many smokers quit successfully without assistance from nicotine replacement products or drug treatment. This is a popular approach.
- ❏ **Nicotine replacement**—Current choices among nicotine patches, and nicotine sprays, and nicotine nasal sprays and nicotine inhalers are discussed a little later in this step.
- ❏ **Medication** available from your doctor that may aid in smoking cessation. This is also discussed a little later in this chapter.
- ❏ Other methods that some have found useful, including **hypnosis** and **acupuncture**.

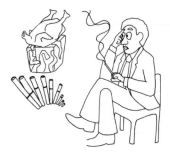

There are TWO ways to quit:
- *Cold turkey.*
- *Tapering off.*

Each of these three questions is independent of the others. You can decide on one or more choices for each.

Many Ways to Quit

In December 1996 the American Lung Association and the Harris organization surveyed smokers about the various methods they have used to try to quit smoking. The most popular method was "cold turkey." But, be careful about this. Simply getting a whim to quit and throwing your cigarettes away rarely leads to quitting for more than a day or two. On the other hand, planning a quit date and then quitting all-or-nothing on that date has worked for many ex-smokers.

Group Cessation Clinics

There's nothing more tried and proven than group smoking cessation clinics. These programs are offered by many hospitals and in many worksites, as well as by voluntary agencies such as the American Lung Association.

The American Lung Association's *Freedom From Smoking*® clinics have helped thousands of smokers to quit successfully. This group approach offers smokers the added benefit of an experienced counselor—the clinic leader—as well as support from a group of peers who are all facing the same problem.

Smokers frequently wonder whether they should try quitting on their own or through a group program. There's no sure answer. But think about how you like to work. If you like to puzzle things out for yourself or, perhaps, build furniture or home devices from kits, then quitting on your own may be for you. On the other hand, if you work well in groups and enjoy meetings—or, at least some of them—then a group program may work for you.

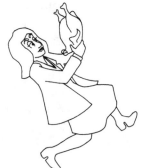

Think you can quit cold turkey?

If you contact a group program, the representatives should be able to describe it for you and answer your questions. If they can't, move on. If they give you the information you need, ask yourself if it sounds like a program that would bring out the best in you. If so, you might give it a try.

GROUP PROGRAMS: QUESTIONS TO ASK

Many smokers who find it difficult to quit on their own join group smoking cessation programs. If you're trying to decide whether a group program is right for you, here are questions to ask when you call for information:

▶ **Is the program convenient?** Find out where it's conducted, what day and time, and how many sessions are involved.

▶ **Is the staff well trained and professional?** Ask who will be leading the group. If a recognized educational, public health or medical organization offers the program, the staff is likely to be well qualified. If the program involves hypnosis, the leader should be a licensed or certified professional in psychiatry, psychology, or social work. If medications are to be used, a physician or other health professional should be involved in screening participants before treatment.

▶ **Does the program provide what you need?** Find out whether the program emphasizes lectures or group discussions. Will you get help with controlling stress and weight gain? Does the program offer continued assistance after the group sessions are over? Be wary if the staff says their program contains a special, foolproof method that will do everything for you.

▶ **What is the success rate of the program?** Research shows that group programs are successful for about 20 to 30 percent of participants. With the addition of nicotine replacement products, hypnosis, and group support to stay off cigarettes, success rates may be increased. A good program follows up on participants for at least three months. Those who are judged successfully quit should be reported as a percentage of all those who participated in the program at least once or twice—including those who dropped out.

▶ **How much will it cost?** Price doesn't necessarily reflect the value of the program. Group programs can cost less than $50 and as much as several hundred dollars. If your employer or health care plan offers a stop-smoking program, it's likely to be less expensive for you.

Group smoking cessation clinics are held year-round in locations throughout the United States. Check the **Resource** section in the back of this book to find the American Lung Association office nearest you.

Nicotine Fading

When you took the **Are You Addicted to Cigarettes?** quiz, did your score indicate that addiction could be a real problem for you during the initial stages of withdrawal? If this makes you hesitant to quit "cold turkey," you may want to consider a technique called **nicotine fading**.

With the nicotine fading method, you reduce your nicotine dose slowly over one to two weeks but still smoke your regular number of cigarettes. You can do this by switching brands. As you know, different brands of cigarettes provide different amounts of nicotine. By switching to cigarettes with lower levels of nicotine, you can gradually bring down your addiction to nicotine *before* you quit smoking. This will help you avoid a steep drop in your nicotine level that can cause strong withdrawal symptoms. You'll then be able to stop smoking more easily when your Quit Day arrives.

If you choose this method, it's important to establish a written plan to fade. There is a tendency to smoke more cigarettes when you reduce their nicotine content.

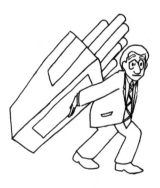

COLD TURKEY TOO TOUGH? Then try to taper off.

Here's how to start fading:

▶ First **check the list below** to find the cigarette brand you are now smoking.

▶ If you're smoking a High nicotine brand, switch to a Medium nicotine brand for one week.

▶ If you're smoking a Medium nicotine brand, switch to a Low nicotine brand for one week.

▶ If you're already smoking a Low nicotine brand, just switch to another Low nicotine brand.

> ### QUICK QUIT TIP
> **You will cut your daily nicotine dose by about a third when you switch to a lower-nicotine level cigarette brand.**

If you do decide to use nicotine fading, be sure to **make a clean break** when you switch. Toss out any cigarettes you are currently smoking. Also stop smoking pipes or cigars and stop chewing tobacco. In addition, **make sure you don't**:

1.. Switch from a high–nicotine brand directly to a low–nicotine brand.
2. Smoke any more cigarettes than you normally do.
3. Inhale more often or more deeply.

NICOTINE FADING
NICOTINE FADING
NICOTINE FADING

Find your brand in the list below, and circle it.

▶ If it's a high-nicotine brand, look in the medium- nicotine brand column and circle your choice of the brand you'd like to fade to.

▶ If your brand is a medium-nicotine brand, look in the low-nicotine brand column and circle the brand you want to fade to.

▶ If your brand is a low-nicotine brand, circle another brand in that same column as your choice of brand you'd like to fade to.

High-Nicotine	*Medium-Nicotine*	*Low-Nicotine*
Alpine	Belair	Benson & Hedges Ultra
American	Benson &	Lights
Austin	Hedges Lights	Bright 100's
Benson & Hedges	Cambridge Lights	Carlton
Best Buy	Camel Lights	Cost Cutter Ultra Lights
Best Value	Capri	Doral Ultra Lights
Cambridge	Century Lights	Famous Value Ultra
Camel	Cost Cutter Lights	Lights
Century 25's	Falcon Lights	Gridlock Ultra Lights
Chesterfield	Famous Value Lights	Merit Ultra Lights
Convoy	Fiesta	Now
Cost Cutter	Kent Golden Lights	Salem Ultra Lights
Craven A	Kim	Triumph

High-Nicotine	Medium-Nicotine	Low-Nicotine
Dunhill	Kool Lights/Mild	True
Eli Cutter	L & M Lights	Vantage Ultra Lights
English Ovals	Lucky Strike Lights	Virginia Slims Ultra Lights
Eve Slim Lights	Magna	Winston Ultra Lights
Famous Value	Malibu Lights	
Gridlock	Marlboro Lights	
Harley Davidson	Marlboro Medium	
Herbert Tareyton	Merit	
Hi-Lite	More Lights	
Kent 100's	Newport Lights	
Kool	No Frills	
L & M	Old Gold Lights	
Lark	Pall Mall Lights	
Lucky Strike	Parliament Lights	
Malibu	Pyramid Ultra Lights	
Marlboro	Raleigh Lights	
Max	Richland Lights	
More	Ritz	
Newport	Royale Lights	
Old Gold	Salem Lights	
Pall Mall	Saratoga	
Philip Morris	Satin	
Players	Silva Thins	
P.M. Blues	True 100's	
Richland	Vantage	
Salem	Viceroy Lights	
Spring	Virginia Slims Lights	
Stride	Winston Lights	
Tall		
Tareyton		

What If Your Brand Isn't on the List?

1. If it's an unfiltered cigarette or if it's a filtered cigarette and does not contain the words "light" or "ultra light," count it as a high-nicotine brand.

2. If it's a filtered cigarette and contains the word "light" or "mild," assume it's a medium-nicotine brand.

3.. If it's a filtered cigarette and contains the words "ultra light," assume it's a low-nicotine brand.

As you proceed with nicotine fading, it's important to remember that this is merely a temporary measure. The main benefits to your health come from quitting entirely. You'll be ready for that with Step 5.

Nicotine Replacement Therapy

If you scored high on the addiction test or if you had a lot of cravings during a previous quit attempt, you may wish to consider using a nicotine substitute product: nicotine gum, nicotine patch, nicotine nasal spray, or nicotine inhaler. Nicotine gum was approved in 1984 by the Food and Drug Administration. The nicotine patch was approved in 1991, nicotine spray in 1996, and the nicotine inhaler in 1997. Research has shown that smokers who use some form of nicotine replacement therapy and participate in a behavior change program like **7 Steps to a Smoke-Free Life** can *double* their chances of quitting for good.

WARNING: YOU MUST QUIT SMOKING COMPLETELY BEFORE STARTING TO USE ANY NICOTINE REPLACEMENT PRODUCT!

People usually develop cravings for things that provide immediate satisfaction, like chocolate or cigarettes. Since nicotine replacement provides nicotine but not the quick nicotine uptake of cigarettes, it's easier to give up nicotine replacement than it is to give up cigarettes. With the patch, the nicotine level in your body stays relatively constant day after day. There is no immediate satisfaction, so there is less craving for a patch. As a result, "quitting" nicotine replacement after you're securely off cigarettes is generally pretty easy.

Nicotine patches, gums, inhalers, and nasal sprays are costly. But during the first year alone, a pack-a-day smoker who successfully quits smoking will more than pay for the medication with the money saved from not buying cigarettes.

Here are some other important things to know about nicotine replacement products:

▶ Nicotine patches and nicotine gum are available over-the-counter. The nicotine nasal spray and nicotine inhaler are currently available only by prescription from a doctor.

▶ They supply small amounts of nicotine that will help relieve

many of the withdrawal symptoms that a smoker may feel
when quitting.

▶ The goal is to be free of both cigarettes and the nicotine substitute within three to six months.

Whether you choose nicotine gum, nicotine patches, or
any other form of nicotine replacement, there's one important
rule to follow:

**You must quit smoking completely before
you use any nicotine replacement.**

That means, *you must not smoke while using these products.*
If you do, you may develop serious side effects caused by an
overdose of nicotine.

Nicotine replacement should not be used by pregnant or
nursing women. With any nicotine substitute, it's always wise
to check with your doctor to see if there are medical reasons
you should not use these products.

Nicotine Gum

Nicotine gum is a drug in gum form, with enough nicotine to
reduce your urge to smoke. The gum releases small amounts of
nicotine, which is absorbed into the body through the mucous
membranes of the mouth. This cuts down on withdrawal symptoms and makes it easier to break the smoking addiction. It tastes
very different from regular gum, because it is a medicine.

You can buy nicotine gum from drug stores, mass merchan-
disers, and supermarkets. Package instructions explain how the
gum is used. Most smokers chew *ten to fifteen pieces of gum a day.*
However, you can have up to thirty pieces. It's important to use as
many as you need to feel comfortable without cigarettes.

QUICK QUIT TIP:

REMEMBER!
With nicotine gum:

Chew it right.
Chew enough.
Chew it long enough.

Use only one piece of gum at a time. Chew it very slowly until you feel a tingle in your mouth. When the peppery taste is present, park the gum between your cheek and gum. When the tingle is gone, chew a few more times to get it back. Then park it again in different parts of your mouth. Repeat this procedure for about thirty minutes to release most of the nicotine. Most of the time nicotine gum is in your mouth, it should be parked. *Do not chew continuously and swallow the saliva as you would with regular gum.* The nicotine from the gum must be absorbed through the mouth—it is ineffective if it's swallowed. The nicotine does not reach the bloodstream if it goes to the stomach, and it can cause heartburn or hiccups.

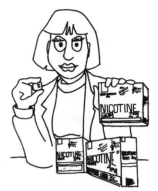

Nicotine Gum

Another important point is: *do not use nicotine gum while you are drinking.* This will wash the nicotine down to the stomach. Wait several minutes after drinking liquid before chewing the gum, and vice versa. This is particularly important if you have been, or will be, drinking acidic beverages such as orange or grapefruit juice because the acidic quality of these drinks changes the "environment" of the mouth and interferes with the amount of nicotine that's absorbed.

Begin using the gum after you quit smoking, and use it every day for at least two to three months after quitting. The first three months are when relapse is most likely to happen. Remember that you must not chew the gum and smoke cigarettes.

As your urges to smoke decrease, you will gradually reduce your use of the gum. Two cautions, however:

1. It's better to use the gum a little longer than to risk a relapse by tapering off the gum too early or too quickly.
2. Even after you stop use of the gum, continue to carry some with you just in case. Better to relapse to the gum than to cigarettes.

Using the Nicotine Patch

The nicotine patch is applied to your skin. Over a prolonged period of time, the nicotine dissolves right through the skin

The nicotine patch, nicotine gum, nicotine inhaler and nicotine nasal spray are temporary aids that can help you make it through the tough times after you've quit smoking.

and enters the body. Nicotine from the patch replaces some of the nicotine you were getting from cigarettes. This can relieve some of the physical symptoms associated with quitting smoking, so you can concentrate on your behavioral and psychological addiction to cigarettes.

You can buy the nicotine patch without a prescription but as always, it's best to check with your doctor to see if the patch is right for you. You may not be able to use the patch if:

- ❏ You are taking certain prescription medicines, or
- ❏ You have cardiovascular disease or certain other health conditions.

Even if you've been told not to use the patch because of a medical condition, you may want to check back with your doctor from time to time, to see if your condition, or the medical advisories, have changed. For example, physicians were initially concerned that nicotine patch use might be dangerous for cigarette smokers who have coronary artery disease. However, a recent study found that the patches are a safe smoking cessation therapy for this group, and may also improve blood and oxygen flow to the heart. Some research has suggested that the patch is safe and effective for teenage smokers, but patch use is currently not advised for people under 18 years of age.

The nicotine patch is safe but, as with any medication, it must be used with caution. Most important, *you should never smoke a cigarette while using the patch.*

Some **side effects** from normal use of the patch can include headaches, dizziness, upset stomach, diarrhea, weakness, or blurred vision. Vivid dreams also may result from an interrupted sleep pattern when you quit smoking.

Used and unused nicotine patches should be kept out of the reach of children and pets.

Some people report a **mild itching or burning** on the skin where the patch is applied, which usually goes away in about an hour. If the irritation continues, you can try moving the patch to a different spot. If it persists, remove the patch and contact your doctor.

Some patches contain more nicotine than others. Some smokers start with the strongest patch. Then after several weeks, you can switch to a medium-strength patch for a few weeks, and possibly a lower-strength patch for the last few weeks. On the other hand, some people prefer the simplicity of a single-strength patch.

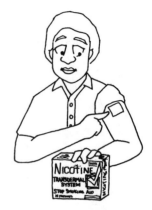

If you do use the nicotine patch, each morning you will apply a new nicotine patch to a clean, dry, nonhairy part of your upper body or upper arm. Don't apply creams on the skin where you will put the patch. Press the patch firmly on your skin. It should stick

Nicotine Patch

to the skin well, allowing you to do all of your usual activities, including bathing.

One brand of the nicotine patch is removed at night, lowering the level of nicotine in the bloodstream, to give the body a rest. Other brands are worn at night as well as during the daytime, and are changed once every 24 hours. When you remove the patch, put a fresh patch on a new area of your upper body. Do not reuse a skin area for at least one week.

The nicotine patch isn't magic. It can't automatically wipe out all your cravings for nicotine. Cravings are diminished and may not last with the patch, but don't expect them to disappear immediately. Even if you still crave cigarettes sometimes while wearing the patch, you are less likely to suffer from several of the major smoking withdrawal symptoms, such as tenseness, irritability, feeling sleepy, and having a hard time concentrating.

Other Products

Nicotine replacement therapy can also be administered via a **nasal spray** or by the newest method, an **oral inhaler**, which was approved by the Food and Drug Administration in 1997.

These products are available only by prescription. Contact your doctor to see if the nicotine spray or inhaler is right for you.

As with all nicotine replacement products, you cannot start

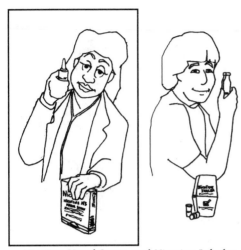

Nicotine Nasal Spray and Nicotine Inhaler

using the nasal spray and the inhaler until you have completely stopped smoking. If you do use nicotine spray or a nicotine inhaler, you must not smoke any cigarettes or use any other form of tobacco, such as cigars, pipes, or chewing tobacco.

The spray delivers nicotine through the nose. The inhaler delivers nicotine into the mouth, which provides a sensation in the back of the throat similar to that produced by cigarette smoke. However, both devices provide nicotine at a lower level than cigarettes, and they do not contain any of the cancer-causing tars and toxins found in tobacco products. For example, ten puffs on the inhaler provides about the same amount of nicotine as one puff on an average cigarette.

With the nicotine **spray and inhaler**, dosage is flexible and can be individualized according to your personal withdrawal symptoms. Both devices deliver nicotine to the bloodstream in a matter of minutes. This fast onset of action reduces nicotine cravings quickly.

Unlike the nicotine patch, gum, and nasal spray, the **nicotine inhaler** has the advantage of satisfying the "hand-to-mouth" ritual smokers miss when they quit. The inhaler consists of a mouthpiece connected to a cartridge containing nicotine. When a smoker puffs on the mouthpiece, the inhaled air becomes saturated with nicotine, which is absorbed through the mucous membranes of the mouth and throat, as occurs with nicotine gum.

This route of absorption isn't the same as that of cigarettes. A majority of the nicotine from a cigarette is absorbed directly into the lungs, which causes a "nicotine spike" that smokers feel almost instantly. It's this spike a smoker gets when taking a puff or a "drag" that contributes to the high addictive properties of tobacco.

Is Nicotine Replacement Unhealthy?

Many people worry that nicotine replacement products are just as bad as smoking cigarettes. They're definitely not. They do not have all the tars and poisonous gases that are found in cigarettes. They provide less nicotine than a smoker would get from cigarettes. And they're designed to help people get off nicotine, not to keep them on nicotine.

Still, it's important to realize that nicotine replacement therapies will not work for everyone. They are not a cure-all. They are just temporary aids that can help you make it through the tough initial withdrawal period after you've quit smoking.

> **Carefully read the directions that come with the nicotine patch, gum, or inhaled products. If you have any questions about their use, ask your doctor or pharmacist.**

What needs to be understood is that nicotine is not the only dangerous element of the smoking habit. Certain moods, times of day, or activities all become strong triggers that make you crave a cigarette. Nicotine replacement isn't a cure for these. That's why anyone who uses the nicotine patch, gum, nasal spray, inhaler, or other products should also make a concerted effort to change their behavior patterns, as described in the rest of this book.

The Non-Nicotine Pill

As this book is being prepared, new medications are emerging to help smokers quit. In fact, there is a new prescription pill that's designed to do just that. Of course, it's still not a magic pill. It doesn't eliminate urges to smoke. Those urges still requires a serious effort to overcome.

This pill is Zyban, the trade name for a sustained-release tablet form of bupropion hydrochloride. This same drug, bupropion hydrochloride, has long been sold as **an antidepressant**, under the trade name Wellbutrin SR. Now it's being marketed as the first non-nicotine prescription treatment for smoking addiction.

How does the pill work for smokers? The drug boosts the body's levels of two "brain chemicals," dopamine and norepinephrine—the same thing that occurs with nicotine. Actions of these chemicals in the brain give people a sense of energy and well being. Nicotine produces the same feelings.

According to the advertisements, using bupropion allows smokers to get the same feeling, while weaning themselves off nicotine. For many people, this helps to reduce withdrawal symptoms and lessens the urge to smoke. But like other nicotine replacement products, the pill should be used in combination with a quit-smoking behavior modification program.

In one study, the non-nicotine pill helped more smokers to quit than the nicotine patch. Using both the pill and the patch was even more effective, but the combination poses the risk of increasing blood pressure.

Zyban is usually taken twice a day—one pill in the morning and one in the early evening. It takes about a week for the pill to reach an effective level in the body. So smokers must start taking the pill *before* they quit smoking. Then you set a Quit Day within one to two weeks after starting treatment. Most smokers then take the pill for a total of seven to twelve weeks.

The non-nicotine pill is available only with a doctor's prescription. It's especially important to get a doctor's advice, because Zyban is certainly not right for everyone. The drug is not recommended for:

▶ Women who are pregnant or breast-feeding
▶ People with a history of eating disorders, such as bulimia or anorexia nervosa
▶ Anyone who is currently taking or has recently taken a monoamine oxidase inhibitor (MAO) medication for depression
▶ People already taking Wellbutrin, Wellbutrin SR, or other medicines that contain bupropion hydrochloride
▶ People who have a seizure disorder, such as epilepsy

Seizures disorders are a special concern. Bupropion is known to cause seizures in approximately 1 out of every 1,000 people taking bupropion hydrochloride. Although this is a small risk, it may be an important factor for people deciding whether or not to use this drug. Other common side effects include dry mouth and difficulty in sleeping.

The Role of Drugs in Quitting

The introduction of bupropion as an aid in smoking cessation is probably a sign of things to come. Better understanding of how smoking influences the brain will probably lead to better drugs to help smokers quit. So, take heart. Try your best now. But also recognize that your efforts to quit are going to receive more types of assistance in the future.

Bupropion also illustrates a major theme of this book, that smoking cessation requires attention to both the biology and psychology of smoking. Bupropion is helpful when used with education programs and support from health professionals or with an intensive self-help program. As with all these assists to quitting, there is still no magic bullet. Bupropion will help smokers quit, but they have to take the first step and continue to work to keep temptations from undermining their efforts.

Alternative Medicine

If patches, sprays, and pills don't appeal to you, you may be more interested in techniques that are often categorized as "alternative medicine."

Two alternative therapies—**hypnosis** and **acupuncture**—have stimulated particular interest as aids to smoking cessation.

Hypnosis is a state of attentive and focused concentration that is induced by the use of "therapeutic suggestion." The hypnotic trance state resembles other forms of deep relaxation. People can't be hypnotized involuntarily and don't follow hypnotic suggestions that are against their wishes. People who desire to be helped are the best hypnotic subjects.

Programs that offer hypnosis as an easy, one-step solution to smoking or other complex problems are without merit. Avoid them!

When employed by psychologists, physicians, and others trained in its use, hypnosis may contribute to smoking cessation. Ask your doctor for a referral, or contact your local or state psychological association for the names of licensed psychologists in your area who practice hypnosis. Like other therapies, though, it's not a magic solution that can be used alone. Hypnosis cannot make you quit or automatically eliminate all your desires to smoke. It should be part of a systematic quit-smoking program.

Acupuncture is an ancient Chinese therapy that involves stimulating specific anatomic points in the body. This regulates or corrects the flow of chi, or energy, in the body, and thus restores health. Puncturing the skin with a needle is the most typical method of acupuncture. As with all other therapies, acupuncture works best for smoking cessation when it's used in combination with a serious effort to quit and a behavior modification strategy to support that effort.

Questions to Ask Your Doctor

Before you start your countdown to quit day, do consider making an appointment with your doctor to discuss your plans. It doesn't matter if the doctor hasn't discussed smoking with you before. Once approached, most doctors will be eager to help you plan a quit program that suits your personal and medical needs.

Your doctor may want to take baseline measurements of your heart rate, blood pressure, and weight. In addition, he or she will determine whether you have any pre-existing medical conditions, such as impaired lung function or chest pains, which might show measurable improvement when you stop smoking. This baseline information will be recorded in your medical chart. That way, you'll have a point of comparison when you return for follow-up visits after you've successfully quit.

Don't forget your dentist, either. Tobacco use has a dramatic effect on the mouth, teeth, and gums. That's why most dentists are eager to help their patients quit smoking. One good way to begin your quit smoking program is to have your dentist clean your teeth, so you'll see some immediate improvement in your appearance right at the start.

Finally, if you are receiving any treatment for depression, anxiety, or other mood disturbances, it's also helpful to check with the person providing this care. Additional counseling or adjustment of medications may help you manage the early stages of smoking cessation.

False Hopes and Phony Solutions

The tobacco companies have brought out several cigarettes they'd like us to believe are safer than regular cigarettes. A product called **Eclipse** burns a piece of charcoal. The smoke from the charcoal passes over beads with nicotine extract on them. The heat from this releases some of the nicotine and flavorings, so the smoker inhales the charcoal smoke, the nicotine, and the flavorings. These devices are lit, and they burn. So you're still inhaling smoke.

The tobacco companies advertise these products with words like "cleaner." They want you to think "safer" but they can't say that because then the government would regulate the product, as Congress requires the regulation of all products that make health claims. There's little doubt that these products—providing inhaled charcoal smoke—are not safe. The American Lung Association and other smoking experts believe **there is no such thing as a safe cigarette**.

Because these devices may reduce the amount of noticeable exhaled and sidestream smoke, they may be deemed acceptable for use in settings where smoking is prohibited—such as workplaces. But smokers using such products may not be helped to quit. In fact, they may wind up smoking more cigarettes to get their usual nicotine.

The tobacco industry has a long history of introducing low-smoke cigarettes, lettuce cigarettes, flavored chewing tobacco, snuff, and other gimmicky devices. Who knows what cigarette manufacturers will come up with next! The real solution is to quit smoking altogether, and not to waste time pursuing the illusion of safe cigarettes.

Time to Set Your Quit Day

You've made a lot of decisions here in Step 3. You have decided whether or not to try nicotine fading or one of the nicotine replacement therapies. Perhaps you've decided to see your doctor to investigate the non-nicotine pill, or alternative therapies such as hypnosis or acupuncture.

"JUSTIN"

Justin had been busy investigating nicotine replacement products. His local drugstore had a special low-price offer on one brand of nicotine patches, so Justin bought a starter kit. He knew that the hours just before lunch and just before the office closed at night were the most stressful times of his workday. So he planned to wear the patch to give himself enough nicotine throughout the day to get by without smoking.

Justin also gave himself an early birthday present: a new pair of running shoes. He used to enjoy jogging but he hadn't run in several years. Once he became determined to get back to a healthier lifestyle, he began doing some light jogging each morning before work. By the time he was ready to quit smoking, he had begun to enjoy the jogging and was seeing results. This helped him control his stress and his weight.

About that birthday—Justin decided not to quit that day as he thought that would put a lot of extra pressure on him. Instead, he set a Quit Date for the first of the month, right after his birthday. On his birthday, as a gift to himself, he spent an hour working on his quitting plans. Choosing a date two and a half weeks from his birthday gave him plenty of time to get ready to quit on the first.

Whatever you've decided so far, you have one more big decision to make. Now is the time to set a date to quit!

Pick a day to quit—about seven to fourteen days from now. Try to choose a day that makes personal sense to you. It should be one that fits your smoking patterns. But it should also reflect the other big things in your life—your family, your work, and how you like to relax and enjoy yourself. For example, many people choose a Monday, so they can start the week off right. Others quit on a Saturday morning so they can have two days to get it down before having to spend a day in the office without cigarettes.

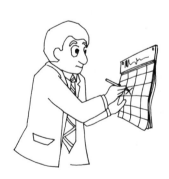

GET READY... Choose a day within the next month to quit

If you smoke a lot at work, you may want to quit over a weekend or maybe over a three-day weekend or holiday, if you have one coming up.

If you are a relaxation smoker—if you like to smoke when you're home on weekends—you might want to quit on a Monday, so you have the whole workweek to get used to it before getting through a Friday or Saturday night without cigarettes.

One clever person recalled that the last time she quit, it really got toughest on the third day. Also, work was worse than being home. So, she quit on a Thursday, so that the tough third day would fall on a Saturday!

Think about it. Make your Quit Date something you feel personally committed to. But whatever day you choose, be sure to:

❑ Mark the date on your calendar. Circle it in red!
❑ Determine to quit on that date.
❑ Spend plenty of time getting used to the idea.
❑ Cross off each day on the calendar as you count down to Quit Day.

Tell yourself that on that day, you will absolutely stop smoking. No fooling around, no kidding yourself, no halfway measures. Just quit. No more cigarettes!

Working up to your Quit Date, you'll proceed with Step 4 to prepare for your Quit Day. You'll learn how to quit right and what to do when you quit. Taking the time to prepare yourself now will help you quit for good!

QUICK QUIT TIP

Psychology at Work

Don't quit *before* your Quit Date! You need to work toward it and get ready for it.

If you're like a lot of smokers we've worked with, this will help you get "geared up" for quitting. You're likely to look forward to your Quit Day and may want to quit a day or two earlier. But don't! Set your Quit Date and work toward it. Then quit!

CHAPTER 8

Step 4
Prepare for
Your Quit Day

Well, you've set a Quit Date and thought about how you are going to quit. You may be feeling, "Am I *really* going to be able to do this?" This chapter will help reassure you that you *can*.

Step 4 covers a lot of specific techniques that will help you to prepare for your Quit Date. It will teach you how to eliminate your strongest urges to smoke before you quit. You'll review Do Power and how it can help you cope with temptations after you quit. You'll learn strategies for getting family and friends to cooperate with you and give you a little encouragement. Then you'll complete a checklist to make sure you're ready. By the time you get to that point, you'll be set to go!

Check Your Pack Track Cards

Getting closer to Quit Day is a good time to look at your Pack Track cards. By now, you should have completed several cards.

Remember how you counted up the check marks under the smiling, sad, and "blah" faces? Now that you have even more cards, can you identify specific moods that seem to trigger your need for a cigarette?

What about the timing of your cigarettes? Do you smoke more at certain times of day, and less at other times? Look to see how much you wanted each cigarette at those times of day.

At this point, definite smoking patterns will be apparent to you. In the rest of Step 4, you'll be using your Pack Tracks to eliminate your strongest urges for cigarettes *before you quit* and to figure out how you can cope with temptations after you quit. For example, you may notice you smoke most of your cigarettes around mealtimes—after breakfast, lunch, and dinner. This tells you that you'll need to focus on activities you can do at these times to reduce your temptation to smoke.

Look to see if you've checked mostly "YES" on your Pack Track cards—if you really have strong cravings for most of the cigarettes you smoke. If so, you may want to decide now that you'll use nicotine replacement after you quit smoking.

Continue to use Pack Track until you quit. It is the single most effective technique for quitting. It will help you identify and plan for temptations after you quit. And, for the very reason it may seem tedious and annoying to do, it breaks up your smoking patterns before you quit, which will make things easier when you do quit.

Eliminating Urges—Eliminating Cues

All around you and all day long, lots of cues tell you it's time to smoke. And these cues are responsible for most of your really strong urges to smoke. Ask yourself, "What's the cigarette that is toughest for me to go without?" Chances are, your answer is something like:

- ❏ "That cigarette with the first cup of coffee in the morning."
- ❏ "Lighting up after getting out of a long movie."
- ❏ "Relaxing with a cigarette after dinner."
- ❏ "Having a cigarette at morning break, after I haven't had one since arriving at work."
- ❏ "Unwinding with a drink and a cigarette when I get home in the evening."

Each of these descriptions centers on a *cue* : the first cup of coffee, getting out of the movie, relaxing after dinner, morning break, and having a drink in the evening. These cues are signals that you and your brain have come to link to smoking—when they happen, you want a cigarette. As a matter of fact, you have linked them so tightly to smoking that they *make you want* a cigarette.

What we are going to describe now is a method to eliminate these toughest cues and, with them, the toughest urges. If you can get rid of some of the cues for smoking *before* you quit, situations in which you've "just got to have a cigarette" will lose some of their power. And you can do it before you quit.

So let's start eliminating cues now. The first step is to identify your strongest cues, the situations in which you *always* smoke.

ARE THERE SITUATIONS WHERE YOU ALWAYS SMOKE?

1. Do you always smoke after dinner? With your morning coffee?
2. Do you always light a cigarette when the phone rings? When your children arrive home from school?
3. Do you always smoke while driving in rush-hour traffic? While driving from errand to errand?

These "always" situations are your strongest external cues for smoking. First, you'll work to eliminate these. Once you feel less need to smoke at the very times you thought you could "never get through without a cigarette," then you'll feel less need in other, less strongly cued situations. Begin eliminating these "always" cues a week or two before your Quit Day. Keep reading to find out how to do it.

Key To Eliminating Cues—The "I Will Never" Rule

To eliminate a cue, you make the decision "I will *never* smoke" when that cue occurs. For instance, if you always smoke when you drink coffee, you must change your pattern so you *never ever* smoke while drinking coffee. This will definitely be hard at first, but if you keep to the "I will never" rule, soon coffee will no longer be a cigarette cue for you.

Here's how to do it.

1. Look back at the list of smoking cues you wrote down in your Pack Track in Step 1 (see page 59). Check off the times or situations when you *always* smoke. Some of these may surprise you. Smoking at these times has been so automatic that you no longer even notice it.
2. Choose two or three "always smoke" cues from your list. Be specific: "In the morning" is too broad. But "sitting at the bus stop in the morning" or "out on an afternoon break at work" are good.
3. Make the commitment: I will *never* smoke when these specific

cues come up. You should still sit at the bus stop—but think about bringing something to read while you wait. You should still continue going out on your break, but maybe you can walk around the block instead of smoking with friends. But *don't* smoke—*ever*!—in these specific situations.

If this seems difficult, try to think of "won't" as "can't." If your doctor told you that you'd have a life-threatening reaction to chocolate, you'd probably find a way to accept that you can't have chocolate.

How Will This Help?

The way the powerful cues have become so strongly linked to smoking is because they occur over and over when you smoke. If you've smoked a pack a day for twenty years and drunk coffee in conjunction with thousands of these cigarettes, that's a lot of times for drinking coffee and inhaling to be linked together. Your body and your mind have learned that, when coffee arrives, nicotine isn't far behind. So, when you drink coffee but then there's no nicotine, you feel a huge urge.

You can eliminate those cues by beginning *not* to smoke when you drink coffee. Just as you learned that coffee and cigarettes go together, you can learn they don't. By using the "I will *never* rule," you can get yourself used to coffee without cigarettes. And, what's really fortunate is that you *can* do this in just the week or so before your Quit Date. Then, when you quit, the urges will be a lot less strong.

Total Separation

For the Eliminating Cues method to work, you must totally separate the cue from the cigarette. If coffee is a cue, it won't work to drink a cup, then have a cigarette, and then drink a second cup. You must wait—say ten minutes—after finishing your coffee before you light a cigarette. And then, don't follow up with another cup of coffee.

What if talking on the phone is your *always* cue to smoke? You must *never* light up while talking on the phone; if you're already smoking when the phone rings, you must either put out the cigarette or just not answer the phone. Remember, the goal is to keep the cue totally separate from smoking.

QUICK QUIT TIP

Hints for Successfully Eliminating Cues

1. **Be consistent.** It's better to choose two or three important cues that you'll *never* smoke with, instead of trying not to smoke with many different cues.
2. **Don't try to quit smoking or even to cut down yet.** Gradually cutting down leads to stronger urges than quitting "cold turkey." So keep smoking for now, but just decide *never* to smoke in connection with the cues you have chosen. You can still smoke at other times.

Feelings Can Be Cues

Some cues for smoking are **external**—a cup of coffee, a ringing telephone, a waiting room. But cues can also be **internal**—the thoughts or feelings inside you that trigger your smoking. For example, you may reach for a cigarette when you feel angry, when you're frustrated or uncomfortable, or when you're feeling unsure of yourself.

Sometimes **external** cues for smoking are easier to recognize than **internal** cues. As you stop smoking in response to external cues, you'll probably become more aware of your internal cues—the feelings and frustrations linked to your smoking. For example, if you stop smoking during a business lunch where you usually would smoke, you'll probably notice feelings such as frustration or boredom that previously had been counteracted by your cigarette smoking. This can help you understand why you always smoked during business lunches.

Keep track of the feelings and frustrations that are cues for your smoking habit. Later on, we'll talk about other ways besides smoking to cope with these feelings. Knowing which feelings really hit your cigarette button will help you spot the ones to work on.

But you can also eliminate your internal cues. For example, if sadness is a big cue for you, make a point of saying, "I will never smoke when I am feeling sad." Then, by the time you get to your Quit Date, feeling sad will not be such a strong cue for smoking. You may still feel sad, but at least it will no longer be a cue to smoke.

Eliminating your strong cues before you quit will mean fewer strong urges to smoke when your Quit Day comes. This is the real plus of Eliminating Cues. Also, it boosts your confidence. Seeing that you can control your strongest cues will help you get the confidence you need to actually quit smoking.

But that's not all you'll need. Eliminating Cues will decrease urges that make you want that cigarette. Next we'll review how Do Power can help you deal with the temptations to smoke after you quit.

Do Power, Or What Self-Control Really Means

Even though you eliminate your strong cues for smoking, you are still going to have temptations to slip up and smoke. You know what that's about:

If you've ever decided to lose weight only to find that you can't resist a bag of potato chips . . .

If you've ever vowed to use spare time constructively, only to end up staring at the television . . .

If you've ever . . . , then you know even the strongest resolution to change your behavior patterns can be thrown off by temptations.

Chapter 3 explained how it's better not to think in terms of will power—either having or not having enough determination to quit. Instead, focus on Do Power—doing things to control those temptations before they knock you off stride.

The very immediacy or closeness of a temptation makes it hard to resist. It's *relatively* easy not to smoke the cigarettes that you haven't bought. But, it's hard not to smoke the cigarette your friend is offering you at coffee break after a hectic morning. You may forget your goal to have a long life when you're in a situation that tempts you to smoke. Often you just can't resist the short-term pleasure, the desire to have just one.

QUICK QUIT TIP

Not Even a Single Cigarette?

One way in which quitting smoking is especially hard is the need to resist all temptations. A dieter who has a single piece of chocolate cake can get back on the diet. The couple of hundred "forbidden" calories won't make too much differ-ence at the end of the week. But having a couple of ciga-rettes *is* a problem. Not always, but usually it leads to relapse. So you do need to avoid *all* cigarettes. It's hard, but one thing you'll find almost all ex-smokers agree on: in the long run, it's "easier to have none than one."

Sounds hopeless? It's not. Remember the essence of Do Power:

▸ Anticipate temptations.

▸ Use Creative Problem Solving to keep the temptation from get ting too close and to keep yourself from being able to yield to its temporary allure.

▸ Do things—follow through with the strategies you created. Use them!

Our creativity ahead of time can be a match for temptation. And, any strategy that blocks momentary temptations or that keeps you from yielding to the temporary urge will increase your self-confidence and help you get to the long-term goal of enjoy-ing life without cigarettes.

Anticipating Temptations

Go back over your Pack Track records. Think about the situations in which you are likely to be tempted. There are a number of ways to approach them. Look at the moods you indicated: anxi-ety, sadness, or happiness. Times when you are especially anx-ious or feeling blue are likely to be especially tempting.

There may also be some situations which don't occur too often, but when they do, oh boy. You are likely to say to your-self, "I'll just hope that doesn't happen." Don't hope—use Do Power. Specify those "oh boy" situations and start making plans for how you are going to handle them.

Use the **Work Sheet for Do Power** on pages 98-99 to help you target your temptations and plan your responses.

Planning Strategies

After specifying your temptations, you need to think of specific things you will do to keep each from getting to you. Here are some questions to ask to help you come up with good strategies:

▸ "How can I avoid the temptation altogether?"

- ▶ "If I can't avoid it, how can I weaken the temptation when I'm in the situation?"
- ▶ "What can I do ahead of time to reduce my urge when tempted?"
- ▶ "When tempted how can I limit my ability to give in to the temptation?"

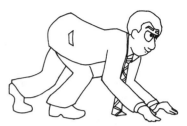

*GET SET...Rearrange
your habits*

Remember to be creative and to get specific in answering these questions. Specific strategies that make sense for you are the best **Do Power.**

Here are some examples to help your creative juices:

Alter Your Environment

- ▶ Get rid of all cigarettes, ashtrays, lighters, and matches.
- ▶ Avoid bars or other places where a lot of people smoke.
- ▶ For a couple of weeks, don't go to lunch or coffee breaks with friends who smoke.

Prepare Yourself

- ▶ Have Creative Alternatives available—sugar-free gum, low-calorie snacks, etc.
- ▶ Plan an enjoyable activity and start it before the temptation occurs—for example take a walk after dinner.

Engineer Your Social World

- ▶ Tell a lot of people that you've quit cigarettes.
- ▶ Make clear to your smoking friends that you don't want them to give you a cigarette—most relapse cigarettes come from a friend.
- ▶ Tell a friend about an upcoming temptation and ask them to give you some encouragement in the situation—say, just before a tense meeting.

Promote Your Goal

- ▶ Rehearse your reasons for quitting.
- ▶ Promise yourself something you enjoy—a movie or dinner at a favorite restaurant—for getting through the first week.
- ▶ Get involved in activities that don't go with smoking— exercise, meditation.
- ▶ Imagine yourself as you'd like to feel, enjoying favorite activities without smoking.

Reduce the Appeal of Temptations
▶ Think about the harmful things cigarettes do to you.
▶ Think about the diseases you're concerned about getting if you go back to smoking.

As these examples show, your Do Power doesn't depend on "inner strength." It rests on how well you anticipate temptations and how creatively you act to change them.

WORK SHEET FOR DO POWER

What situations tempt you to smoke? List and describe them here.
Write in the Do Power strategies you can use to block these temptations.

TEMPTATION #1
Where: _____
When: _____
With whom: _____
Reason for urge: _____
Strategies for #1:
a) _____
b) _____
c) _____

TEMPTATION #2
Where: _____
When: _____
With whom: _____
Reason for urge: _____
Strategies for #2:
a) _____
b) _____
c) _____

TEMPTATION #3
Where: _____
When: _____
With whom: _____
Reason for urge: _____
Strategies for #3:
a) _____
b) _____
c) _____

Temptation #4

Where: _____

When: _____

With whom: _____

Reason for urge: _____

Strategies for #4:

a) _____

b) _____

c _____

Too Much Work?

"This Do Power sounds like a lot of boring work. Who wants to make lists of temptations and strategies for fighting them? I'll just do my best and hope for the best."

Yes, Do Power does require some effort in advance. You probably already have enough things in your life that require planning. You don't need another opportunity to show how clever you can be.

But remember: Quitting smoking is the most important and one of the hardest things you'll do all year. Give it the attention that it—**and you**—deserve!

Cooperation and Encouragement

You're the one who puts a cigarette in your mouth and smokes it, but others can still play an important role in your smoking habit—and in your efforts to quit. Quitting goes a lot more smoothly and is more successful if you have cooperation and encouragement from your family and friends.

> **QUICK QUIT TIP**
>
> **Cooperation and encouragement from your friends and family are critical to your success in stopping smoking.**

Can you think of three people you can use for your quit team? Try to choose:

▶ One person from your immediate family

▶ One person from work

▶ One person from your circle of friends

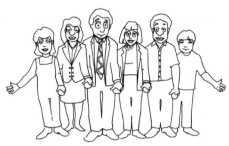

Get a friend or your husband or wife to quit with you

A spouse or family member can be a help when you quit. They will care a lot whether you quit and may be willing to cooperate in ways that can really help. But, sometimes their caring can get in the way. If you want to discuss doubts or a slip, they may react with anxiety more than with encouragement. So also identify at least one nonsmoking person you can turn to if you just want to speak with someone who isn't so anxious for you to quit.

If you know any **former smokers** who have successfully quit, try to recruit them for your team. Ex-smokers have "walked in your shoes" and know what you're going through—and what benefits you'll gain from quitting for good. The success they've had in conquering cravings, overcoming withdrawal symptoms, and handling stressful situations without cigarettes can make ex-smokers a valuable source of support and guidance for you.

QUICK QUIT TIP

Quit with a Friend?

Some people try to quit with a friend or a spouse or partner. This has some strong points. Your teammate will be going through the same thing you are. He or she will know what you are trying to do and how you are trying to do it. A buddy says, "We are both quitting smoking. Let's hold each other to it, and have fun at the same time."

But there can be downsides too. Unfortunately, people who quit together often relapse together. If you are thinking of quitting with a friend, make sure you feel secure he will not drag you down with him if he has trouble. If he relapses, will you feel you need to as well in order not to make him feel bad? Would he feel you are dropping him if you spend a little less time with him or refuse to smoke when you are together?

Definitely do **not** talk other people into quitting with you. If they truly want quit with you, it may be a big help. But if they are just going along with your campaign, they are likely to be a weight you don't need.

You may feel awkward and uncomfortable asking for encouragement and cooperation. Tell yourself it's okay to get help from other people. They can't do it for you, but they can make things a little easier for you. And you'll probably be surprised at the good response you'll get. Many people who you might never have guessed had been smokers have quit smoking. They'll be glad to share their experiences. Also, people at home and at work who don't like being exposed to your cigarette smoke will be happy to encourage your decision to quit.

QUICK QUIT TIP

How Solid Is Your Support?

What if your friends and family are smokers and don't really want to support you? They may feel uncomfortable helping you to do something they haven't been able to do themselves. You will need to separate your goals from your feelings about them. They probably can't give you too much of the encouragement you deserve if they feel badly about their own smoking. What you can do is ask them to cooperate with your efforts in very specific ways. Particularly, think about times when it would really help if they didn't smoke around you, like after dinner or in the car. Try negotiating some modest deals with them. And remember, cooperation needs to be a two-way street, so be prepared to have something you can do for them—maybe by not bragging about your success!

Remember, you deserve cooperation! You are about to carry out one of the hardest and most important things you can do for yourself and the people around you. You are now on your way to a smoke-free *you* and a smoke-free *life*. It will be a better life for you and the people close to you. So don't expect any less cooperation from friends and family than for any other very hard and very important task.

> "I wanted to have a lot of support people. I chose someone at my office, and I chose someone in my family—my sister—and I chose a friend of mine."
> —Barbara, age 49

Tell Your Team How to Help You

Some people may hesitate to help you simply because they're not sure what they can do. It's up to *you* to tell them! If you want them to call you, tell them. If you don't want calls, let them know that, too.

What are some other ways people can help you? They can:

▶ Hear you out when you're tempted to smoke
▶ Suggest methods for getting past the urge
▶ Stop by to see you—or call you—on days you know will be hard for you
▶ Help explain your needs to your spouse
▶ Be available just to listen to you complain about how awful it is—or brag about how well you're doing!

QUICK QUIT TIP

Style, Not Substance

Some people say they aren't into getting cooperation and encouragement from others. What they are really saying is that they don't want "gushy" or "flowery" support from others. That's fine. Some people want roses and a singing telegram—some want a brief "Good job." Think about what style of encouragement and cooperation you want and ask for it. But don't make the mistake of thinking you need to do it all alone. The only one we know who does it all alone is the Marlboro Man—and he's still smoking!

Think of your own personal situation. What would be most helpful to *you*? For example, some people always have strong cravings for cigarettes in social situations. One man who had just given up smoking was going to a party where he knew his desire to smoke would be tremendous. He asked his friends in advance not to give him cigarettes that night, even if he begged and pleaded.

One option you might consider to let key people know how serious you are is to put your request in writing. You can ask your friends and family to agree to support you *throughout* your attempt to quit, and just generally "be there"—even if you get crabby during the first week or two after quitting. Then list specific actions that are especially important to you.

INFORMATION FOR YOUR SUPPORT PEOPLE

Copy this letter and send one (or e-mail it) to each of your support people, or use this as a model for letters you compose.

Dear _____,

I need your help to stop smoking! Doctors have shown that friends and family can be a big help to someone who wants to stop smoking. Here are some things you can do to help me stop smoking for good.

1. Be positive. Tell me you're glad I've stopped smoking.
2. Please put up with me if I'm crabby or cranky the first few days after I stop smoking. While I'm giving up cigarettes, I may be on edge. This will go away soon.
3. Ask me how things are going from time to time.
4. Make a change for the better yourself—like always wearing seatbelts if you've been negligent about that.
5. Reward and praise me. Rewards don't have to be presents—a note or a hug will do.
6. Don't tempt me. It's hard enough without seeing and smelling cigarettes. It'll be tough if you offer me a cigarette or smoke in front of me.
7. Don't nag. Be understanding.
8. If I slip up, tell me not to give up.

Here are some other things you can do:

_____

_____

Thank you for helping me to stop smoking. It means a lot to me!

Sincerely,

_____ (signature of smoker)

Another way to let key people know how you would like their encouragement or cooperation is to talk with them about it. (You'd probably do this for other important things you were trying, right?) Ask them to spend a few minutes with you on this. Use the following as a starting point.

> "I felt sort of hesitant to ask people to help me—particularly someone at work—because I thought, oh, you know, they may not want to. But the fact was he was very happy to help me. I really think most people do want to help you stop smoking. It's just a question of asking."
> —Kenneth, 28

HELPING OTHERS QUIT SMOKING

Here are some "talking points" you should discuss with support team members.

For the Quitter:

1. What does it mean to you for some one to "be there"?
2. When will you need people to put up with you—when you're crabby or cranky the first few days after you stop smoking? Or in the weeks following, when it's no longer a novelty?
3. How would you like others to cooperate with your efforts? Are there specific times you'll need them to give you an assist?
4. Do you want to be asked how things are going or how you're doing? About how often or when?
5. Are there some prizes or rewards that you would like when you've been successful? Are there some that would be fun for both you and your family member or friend?

For the Friend or Family Member:

1. Be positive. Tell them how glad you are they've stopped smoking.
2. Reward and praise them. Rewards don't have to cost much— they can be "flowery" or simple, whatever suits your style.
3. Don't nag. Focus on how hard they are trying and how much you recognize that.
4. Understand that they may want to talk about wanting a cigarette or having a slip. This does **not** mean they don't really want to quit.
5. Don't tell them how to feel. Accept and try to understand how they *are* feeling.
6. Don't tell them what to do. Ask them what they are thinking of doing and try to get them to think about the pros and cons.
7. If they slip up, encourage them not to give up.

In fact, it's a good idea to discuss these issues with other people, too—your spouse, friends, and coworkers. Explain to them that you'd like them to be willing to listen when you ask for their time. If you'd rather that they let you bring the subject up first, tell them.

Working Together

If you're quitting with a friend or just lining up some encouragement for your own efforts, be sure to have phone numbers handy. A telephone call can give you or your friend just the needed boost to help lift your mood and keep you from smoking. You and your friend may want to call each other, or get together, at a certain time each day. Remember, quitting smoking is important, so think about scheduling specific times to meet or talk on the phone, just as you would a business appointment.

Low Moods, Anxiety, and a Kind Word

When people quit smoking, they sometimes feel low, sorry for themselves, lonely, and deprived. That's when the encouragement of family or friends can be particularly helpful. If you think you are going to be feeling sorry for yourself for a couple of days, tell others ahead of time and discuss what you can plan to combat it.

Often people will feel they don't know what to say. Some well-intentioned things people say may be misinterpreted as "nagging" or "bossy." So tell your friends anything you think is important to know about you and what kind of "helpful suggestions" you can deal with.

An Encouragement Plan

It's a good idea to set up a specific plan with key people. Use the form below to help you commit to following through. Be creative. Let it change, as needed. But have a plan. You wouldn't want your community to hire firemen after your house started to burn! Try to keep in contact with someone on your team at least every 48 hours. With frequent contact, you can stick to your plan.

A WORK PLAN FOR QUITTING

*Use this form to create a support plan for you
and your team members to follow.*

We will maintain contact in the following ways:_____
_____
_____

When_____ is tempted to smoke, she/he will contact you in the
following ways: _____
_____
_____

_____ will cooperate by remembering to: _____
_____
_____

_____ will cooperate by remembering not to:_____
_____
_____

What's really important for_____ to remember in getting cooperation and encouragement is: _____
_____
_____

What's really important for _____ to remember in *giving*
cooperation and encouragement is: _____
_____

Plan Your Alternatives to Smoking

The key to quitting is to plan ahead. So far, you've made plans
for dealing with temptations and you've planned to recruit support people. Now you've got to **plan specific activities** that
can take the place of smoking.

"That's impossible! Nothing could possibly take the place of smoking." Yeah,
that nicotine is good stuff and you've gotten pretty good at using it. Stirring sticks
and carrot strips are not really going to
give you that rush. But at least you'll have

**"I called a friend when I had trouble avoiding a cigarette. I asked her to talk me out of it or keep me company to distract me. It worked!"
—Jonathan, age 36**

something to do to distract yourself and to keep yourself busy, wherever you are, when you feel the urge to smoke.

You'll definitely need **things to do with your hands and mouth**. Some people suck on stirring sticks, or fiddle with paper clips. Others go for a brisk walk. Many people find that a few deep breaths work best. Calling up one of your support people can also help. Or sit down and write a letter.

Chewing gum can help, too. If you're using nicotine gum, be sure to have several pieces with you at all times.

These activities may not discourage urges but at least they"ll give you something to do instead of just sitting there, craving that cigarette.

QUICK QUIT TIPS

A Survival Kit

Here's something to do before you stop smoking:
Pack a survival kit of things you can use to keep your hands and mouth busy whenever you're tempted to smoke. Keep your survival kit with you at all times.

Suggested contents include:

▶ Stirring sticks   ▶ Cinnamon sticks
▶ Sugarless gum   ▶ Rubber bands
▶ Sugarless candy   ▶ Paper clips
▶ A ball to squeeze   ▶ A pencil to hold

Keeping busy is also important to keep your mind off smoking. Plan ahead to get together often with friends, schedule outdoor activities, and stock up on magazines and videos. If you don't have a hobby, this is a good time to start one. You may also need to spend more time with people who don't smoke. So try going places where smoking isn't permitted.

Look back at **Blockbuster #4** in Chapter 3 for a long list of other Creative Alternatives to smoking. There are many, many activities to choose from. The key is to plan your alternatives ahead of time, so they'll be ready and available to you when temptations hit.

Q U I C K   Q U I T   T I P

Mind Game Rehearsal

One way to prepare yourself in advance is to imagine yourself tempted in a "trigger situation" where you're really likely to crave cigarettes. Then imagine carrying out the Do Power or Creative Alternative plan you've developed. Imagine yourself going through each step.

Different Strokes for Different Folks: For some people, this may sound like fun. For others, it may sound corny. But, whether it's fun or corny, it works. As with a lot of what we've talked about, the key is to be specific. Really imagine yourself carrying out each step of your plan for keeping that temptation from getting the better of you.

An Example: You're at a big wedding. You're talking with an old friend you haven't seen for years. He takes out a pack of cigarettes, opens it up, and offers you one. What happens next?

Right! You smile and say, "No thanks. I've quit smoking." Your friend is supportive and asks what finally made you decide to do it. You end up telling him your reasons for quitting and feel your mood improve.

Don't Forget Diet and Exercise

Of course, you may want to drink or eat as an alternative to smoking. Food and drink can indeed be a convenient and tempting substitute. Also, you may find yourself hungry more frequently after you give up cigarettes. Quitting also can cause metabolic changes that lead to an initial weight gain.

Be prepared! Here's another area where Do Power's advance planning pays off:

▶ Keep a supply of healthy snacks like fruit or veggie sticks on hand.

▶ Drink a large glass of water or a low-calorie beverage whenever you get the urge to smoke.

▶ Instead of eating and drinking, try exercising —even just going for a walk around the block—to keep your mind off smoking.

And remember, just because you're depriving yourself of cigarettes doesn't mean you have to deprive yourself of your favorite
foods. You are likely to be concerned about weight gain, but
you don't have to eliminate all the foods that you enjoy. Try to
eat a well-balanced diet. The best foods to include are fruits and
vegetables, beans, whole grain breads, rice, pastas—the low-
sugar, low-fat, low-calorie foods. If you fill up on these foods,
you're less likely to be tempted by candies and pastries.

Exercise helps, too. If you haven't exercised much before,
talk to your doctor about a sensible exercise program. There's
no need to become a "jock" overnight, but there are many good
reasons to start a regular regimen of brisk walking, bicycle riding, swimming, or any other physical
activity you enjoy.

Exercise will increase your metabolic rate and help your body burn
extra calories. Exercise also helps
reduce tension and stress, which will
make you feel more relaxed and alert.
All of these benefits can be a big help

> "My doctor told me that the best
> thing I could do was just walk—
> at a pretty good pace. And that
> was fine with me, because I'm
> not really big into exercise
> anyway, and anybody can walk."
> —Sylvia, age 66

to you in quitting smoking and minimizing weight gain.

Focusing on diet and exercise is a healthy part of your quitting plan. But don't get so busy with these concerns that you
lose sight of your real goal. Remember, your chief priority is quitting smoking!

Time to Answer the Big Question

At this point, you're more than halfway through the **7 Steps To
A Smoke-Free Life** program. You've completed Steps 1, 2, and
3, and now you're finishing Step 4. So now it's time to answer a
big question:

**If someone walked up to you right now and asked, "Are
you ready to quit smoking?" what would you say?**

Do you feel that you can deal with the roadblocks that have
held you back? Do you have more confidence in yourself? Here
are some important questions to help you decide:

ARE YOU READY TO QUIT SMOKING?

*Circle **YES** or **NO**.*

1. Do I believe that smoking is dangerous to my health?
   YES   NO

2. Besides health reasons, do I have other personal reasons for quitting smoking?
   YES   NO

3. Am I committed to trying to quit even though it may be tough at first?
   YES   NO

4. Is quitting smoking a #1 priority for me?
   YES   NO

5. Are my family, friends, and coworkers willing to help me quit smoking?
   YES   NO

6. Have I planned specific Do Power strategies for handling temptations?
   YES   NO

7. Will I be patient with myself if I backslide?
   YES   NO

If you answered "YES" to most of these questions, you're ready to quit.

But if going through these questions makes you wonder, you've got some more work to do to get ready for your Quit Date:

▶ Go back and skim through the beginning chapters of this book.

▶ Focus again on your personal reasons for quitting, and on the health risks of continuing to smoke. Re-read your **Top 5 Reasons** card.

▶ Reconsider the barriers and "back doors" that are still holding you back. Review the Blockbusters that can break through those barriers.

▶ Write out some additional confidence-building statements.

Are You Really Ready?

Okay, the plan is for you to quit on your Quit Date. But, maybe you are thinking that you are really not ready. Remember the key fact: the average *successful* quitter relapses a few times before staying smoke-free. So making attempts and learning from them is part of the program, not a failure.

The fact that you are reading this book means that you want to quit. Just thinking about quitting is an important first step in the right direction. It may take you a while before you're ready to make the quit, but don't get discouraged. By doing what you've already done, you've definitely moved closer to success in the future. If you decide to hold off for a while, talk with several friends or coworkers who have already quit smoking. Let them tell you firsthand what strategies they used to break the habit, and how much better they feel now that they're non-smokers. There is evidence all around you that people *can* stop smoking. More than 46 million Americans have quit.

Also check the list of organizations included in the Resource section of this book. The American Lung Association and many local hospitals offer group programs or individual counseling to help people quit. Or, you may want to discuss it with your doctor to give your plan a boost.

Of course, go back through the first three Steps and see what seems to click for you in terms of making you feel you're working on something worthwhile. When you're ready, set another Quit Date and then go through Step 4 again. Then, chances are good that you'll answer "Yes" to the questions in the *Are You Ready to Quit Smoking* test and be ready for Step 5, your Quit Day.

CHAPTER 9

Step 5
Quitting

Your Quit Day is one of the most important days of your life. You've gotten ready to quit. You've thought about it. You understand your smoking habit and you know why you want to quit. You've learned many things to help you make it over the next few weeks without smoking.

You *can* do it! You're well prepared and ready to be smoke-free for life! You'll be the nonsmoker you want to be.

The Day Before

It's important to quit with determination, not with a whimper. The following sections are for the day or so before your Quit Date. They'll help you get your energy and confidence focused on the big change you're making.

Are You Getting Nervous?

Quitting is a big step, a major change in your life. It's natural to be worried and nervous. Try to think of yourself as being more geared up and excited than worried and nervous.

Look again at your Top 5 Reasons for Not Smoking. Think about why you want to do this. Make sure you are clear on *your* reasons for quitting.

To make you feel more confident, review your plans now and you'll realize you really have arranged to make this a success. Ask yourself: How have you done in eliminating the cigarettes associated with your strongest urges? If you've done well, your quitting will be a lot easier because those killer cigarettes won't be half as big an issue as you had feared.

▶ What Creative Alternatives do you have lined up to take the place of cigarettes?

▶ What are your Do Power strategies for fighting temptations after you quit?

▶ What plans do you have for getting cooperation and encouragement from your friends and family?

Reviewing points these should make you confident you are prepared. You probably won't feel giddy or cocky. You still are going to give up something that you'll really miss and it will be hard. But you should feel determined and well-prepared.

Marshaling Resources and Being Good to Yourself

This is a good time to remember a key point of this book:

Quitting smoking is important and difficult.

You are taking on a big one. So be nice to yourself! Cut yourself some slack. If you can become smoke-free in the next few weeks, you don't need to do anything else to prove you're a hero.

▶ Plan an easy day for your Quit Date. You may want it to be a busy one, so you have lots of distraction. Or you may want it to be a relaxing one. Regardless, try to make it a day with the fewest demands possible.

▶ Remind your family and friends that you're counting on their cooperation and encouragement in the next week or two. You might want to ask someone you think is really understanding to spend some time hearing you out about your feelings.

▶ The next section talks about rewarding yourself. If you haven't planned some reward for the first day or two, you should consider it. Rewards aren't the reason you quit, but they can help show yourself that what you're doing is important and that it's worth a little enjoyment.

The Best Reward

Quitting is its own best reward. But you deserve many other rewards for not smoking.

Rewards don't have to be big or expensive—they can even be free. But reward yourself with things you care about or like.

Here's a list of rewards other people have used. Add to the list with some special rewards of your own.

PAYOFFS FOR QUITTING

▶ Buy a new compact disc, tape, or magazine.

▶ Stay in bed late.

▶ Get a new hairstyle for the new you.

▶ Buy new running shoes or exercise equipment.

▶ Call a friend or family member.

▶ Get tickets to a sports event or concert.

▶ Spend extra time on a hobby.

▶ Go to a movie or rent an old favorite.

▶ Buy yourself some flowers.

▶ Have someone else do the chores for a week.

▶ Set aside time to do what you want.

▶ Others: _____

▶ _____

Identify some rewards that make sense for you. This is a little like getting encouragement from your friends. What seems like a great idea to one person may seem silly to someone else. But, we all do better with rewards. You should also plan a series of rewards for milestones in your quitting. Think about what will be the big moments when you will know you have made progress, and plan a reward for each. The Reward Worksheet below will help with this.

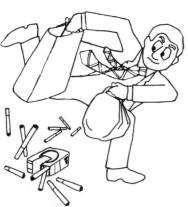

GO... When the date arrives, boost off with a positive attitude.

REWARD WORKSHEET

First day or two:

When I have gone _____ without smoking I will reward myself
with: _____

3 days to one week:

When I have gone _____ without smoking I will reward myself
with: _____

First 2 weeks:

When I have gone _____ without smoking I will reward myself
with: _____

First month:

When I have gone _____ without smoking I will reward myself
with: _____

3 months:

When I have gone _____ without smoking I will reward myself
with: _____

6 months:

When I have gone _____ without smoking I will reward myself
with: _____

Key Temptations

You also should plan some rewards for coping successfully with key
temptations:

When I have gone through _____ without having a cigarette, I will
reward myself with: _____

When I have gone through _____ without having a cigarette, I will
reward myself with: _____

One way to make the rewards you identified more meaningful is to buy them with the money you'll save by quitting. At
a few dollars day, you'll soon have a nice little account there. Also,
using the money you've saved to buy rewards for yourself will
provide another reason for you to quit!

The Nonsmoking Payback!

Every day you go without smoking, you're saving money. Get a big clear glass jar or clear plastic container and plan to put what you would have spent on cigarettes each day into the jar. Watching those coins and dollars pile up can be a wonderful reminder of the benefits of being a nonsmoker.

HOW MUCH WILL YOU SAVE BY NOT SMOKING?

Here's one way to figure out how much money you're going to save. Just multiply 365 days by what you spend each day on cigarettes:

$$365 \times \underline{\hspace{3cm}} = \underline{\hspace{3cm}}$$
(daily cost)   (yearly savings)

Contracts and Commitment

A more formal way to use the reward system—which provides added motivation for many smokers—is to commit yourself in writing to a specific reward for a specific accomplishment.

In other words, you may want to sign a **written** contract like the one on the next page. Use it as a model or tear it out and make it your own. The contract puts in writing your commitment to be good to yourself for your progress in quitting. Many people—perhaps you're included here—have trouble giving themselves the credit or a little praise or reward when they've done something well. You can look at the contract as a way of holding yourself to your word to be good to yourself.

Remember, you don't have to make a contract. If it seems too structured for you, don't bother with it. Of course, you could also alter the contract according to your own preferences. Whether or not you write out a contract, though, it's important to plan some rewards for yourself when meeting your goals. Whether it's down on paper and signed or just in your head, make sure it's clear to you so that it can motivate you in the days to come.

FREEDOM FROM SMOKING CONTRACT

I, _____, am committed to not smoking for the next _____ days. When I am successful in not smoking until _____ o'clock on _____, I will give myself the following reward: _____.

Signed _____

Witnessed _____

Start Spreading the News

Before you quit, it's a good idea to tell your friends, your family, and your coworkers that you are going to be smoke-free as of tomorrow. Even those whom you are not going to look to for support should still know. The more people around you who know you are quitting, the less you will want to give in to temptations. Also, many people will want to help you quit and will be happy to give you some encouragement.

Quitting is an important step for you, but there are sure to be some people who won't understand what you're going through and may not make it easy for you. There are a few bad apples in every barrel. So don't let anyone put you down. Rehearse in your mind how you'll reply to negative comments.

RESPONSES TO CHALLENGES

"When I told my neighbor I planned to stop smoking, she said, 'Oh sure! You've stopped many times.' "

So then I said . . .

▶ "Sure, I went back to smoking before. But doctors say most quitters need to try a few times before they quit for good so I guess I was just practicing"

▶ "Well, you can be skeptical, but at least give me some encouragement. Okay?"

▶ "Yes, but this time I'm in training for the Olympics and my coach won't let me smoke."

▶ "Yes, I know I may not get it this time, but I've been working pretty hard to get ready and I think I have a good chance."

▶ [Your choice]

Nicotine Replacement

If you're planning to use nicotine gum, nicotine patches, or any other form of nicotine replacement, be sure you have these items on hand, so they'll be ready for you to use. Do read the instructions thoroughly, but don't start using any of these products until you eventually stop smoking. Remember:

**You must quit smoking completely before
you use any nicotine replacement.**

If you don't follow this important instruction, you could develop serious side effects caused by an overdose of nicotine.

If your doctor has prescribed Zyban (the non-nicotine pill) or any other medication, be sure that you are taking this medication as directed, so that it will be at an effective level in your body on your Quit Day.

Practice Your Creative Alternatives

In preparation for your Quit Day, today is also a good day to get out the **Survival Kit** you packed. (See Step 4, page 107.) Be sure you have a good supply of sugarless candy and gum, drink-stirring sticks, and any other items you can turn to when you feel tempted by cigarettes.

Spend some time thinking about when you will use the Creative Alternatives you have identified for yourself. You might even pick a couple of situations during the day when you would normally have a cigarette, such as while waiting for the elevator or talking on the phone. Instead, try one of your Creative Alternatives.

The work sheet below may be helpful to you in planning your Creative Alternatives. It's intended to be small enough to fit in your wallet or pocket.

> "It helps when you realize how resilient your body is when you do decide to quit. Unless serious chronic illness has already set in, most of the damage you have done to yourself will reverse itself.—Josh, age 35

ALTERNATIVES WORKSHEET

Situation That Tempts Me   *Creative Alternative*

———————————————   ———————————————

———————————————   ———————————————

———————————————   ———————————————

———————————————   ———————————————

———————————————   ———————————————

Relieve Your Stress with Relaxercise

Simply reviewing all your preparations and thinking about the challenge ahead will make most people a bit tense and nervous. Remember Relaxercise from Chapter 3? Don't reach for a cigarette! Instead, figure out a time today you can use the Relaxercise. Even if you haven't been practicing it, you can start today—it will be a help in the weeks ahead.

For quick review, here's how to do Relaxercise:

- ▶ Sit down anywhere and close your eyes
- ▶ Think about something that makes you feel good.
- ▶ Relax your shoulders. Close your mouth. Inhale slowly and as deeply as you can. Keep your shoulders relaxed.
- ▶ Hold your breath while you count to four.
- ▶ Exhale slowly, letting out all of the air from your lungs.
- ▶ Slowly repeat these steps five times.

Plan to *Relaxercise* at least once every day at least until you feel secure that you are done with cigarettes. You may want to do it more often in the next couple of weeks. For many, it is a great Creative Alternative to smoking.

READ THIS THE NIGHT BEFORE QUIT DAY

- ▶ Be good to yourself. Eat a food you like. Watch a video. Take a long bath.
- ▶ Get a good night's sleep and be well rested for the big day ahead!

Tonight you'll have your last cigarette! Either before you smoke it or when you've finished, here's what to do:

▶ Get rid of all the cigarettes in your house.

▶ Look for any cigarettes that may be in the pockets of your clothes, in the cupboards, in your office, in your car. *Get rid of all of them now!* Run water on them or crumble them up, if that helps.

▶ Get rid of your ashtrays, lighters, and matches.

▶ Review your Top 5 Reasons for Not Smoking. Reflect on what they mean to you. An addition you make tonight may be especially meaningful and helpful in the days to come.

▶ Read over A Fresh Start to Life Without Cigarettes below and plan how you'll organize tomorrow morning.

▶ Try to go to sleep feeling good about yourself. You are about to do something that will be hard, but will give you lots of satisfaction for many years to come.

QUICK QUIT TIP
**Read this the night before you quit—
and follow it that first day.**

A Fresh Start to Life Without Cigarettes

This is the big day! You're well prepared and ready to be smoke-free.

To get your day started right, get up right away and head straight for the shower. If you've been accustomed to smoking immediately on waking up, this quick shower will help you start right on your first day as a nonsmoker. If you're going to use nicotine gum or the nicotine patch, now's the time to start. Be sure to follow the directions on the package or in the guidelines given to you by your doctor.

Get dressed and eat your breakfast pretty quickly this morning. If your usual routine is to linger over breakfast coffee with a cigarette, skip the coffee today. Or buy it on your way to work, in a store where no smoking is permitted.

When you're eating lunch, taking a work break, or going out shopping today, choose places where smoking isn't allowed. And for your first few days as a nonsmoker, try to make an effort to spend more time with people who don't smoke. On the other hand, if you are going to be with smokers, tell people ahead of time that you have quit and that they should not offer you a cigarette. If you're with people whom you don't know well, you may feel somewhat uncomfortable with this

---

announcement. But many people will congratulate you. If someone does slip and offers you a cigarette, remember the assertive responses you practiced for saying a firm "No!" to temptation.

Today may be a good time to keep your schedule pretty full, so you won't have time on your hands. Line up some easy chores, favorite magazines, or tasks that must get done right away. That way, if you have even a few minutes with nothing to do, you can immediately keep yourself busy.

Your Quit Day

It's here! You've waited for it, dreaded it at times, maybe surprised yourself by looking forward to it a little, prepared for it. Well, here it is.

If you've done just a portion of all the things this book has recommended so far, you should be ready. So feel confident as you take the big step in this very important accomplishment.

THE ONE WAY QUITTING SMOKING IS EASY

Think about all the difficult things you try to do in life: eating well, staying organized, keeping the pile of bills on your desk to a height of less than ten inches. In a lot of ways, quitting smoking is harder than each of these. But here's one way it's easier:

**Once you put out that last cigarette, you became
an ex-smoker.
You don't have to do anything more!**

In contrast, think about someone who needs to lose twenty pounds. They can work hard for a week, lose three pounds— "just like the doctor ordered," feel great for a moment, and then realize they still have to lose seventeen more! Or think about yourself and exercising, doing the laundry, or paying the bills. You feel great that you got a good workout today, got fresh sheets on all the beds, or got the desk clear. But tomorrow and next week and next month, you'll need to exercise, do the laundry, or pay the bills all over again.

Of course, staying off cigarettes is going to be hard, especially over the next week or so. But, if you can stay off, you've reached your goal. You don't have to do anything more, and you don't have to quit again tomorrow or next week or next month!

This Day is Not Easy

The first day of quitting is tough. You may feel you have little energy to do much else than hold on. I remember the first smoking cessation class I ran about twenty years ago. After about five minutes of the session on Quit Day, I threw my carefully planned outline in the trash. What I needed to do was sit back, and let everyone in the group vent, complain, "get it off their chest"— and sometimes even beg for mercy! And by the end of the session, they had all gotten around to talking about how they still felt determined, knew that "this too shall pass," and, the nicest part of all, started to compliment and encourage one another for the good work they'd done and the confidence they shared.

Q U I C K   Q U I T   T I P

It's All How You Look at It!

Try this—it works for lots of people:
Think of withdrawal symptoms as "recovery symptoms" as the body returns to a normal nonsmoking state.

It's normal to have a hard time today. It doesn't mean there's anything wrong with you. And it certainly doesn't mean that your case is too hard, or that you can't quit. So don't be scared. Be easy on yourself. Treat yourself like the people in that Quit Day session twenty years ago. Let yourself complain and "beg for mercy" a little. Try not to get rattled by the fact that, yes, it is hard. Just as in the group, after a while you'll start to feel better and realize you'll make it. After a few hours without a cigarette—say, making it past morning coffee break—you'll start to feel like complimenting yourself. You won't feel too confident, but you will feel, "Hey, I just may be able to do this thing!"

Symptoms of Recovery

Quitting smoking brings on a variety of physical and psychological symptoms. Reviewing your 5 Reasons for Quitting and all your preparation can help you feel up to the challenge, but there's no way to avoid all of the physical effects. But what can help is simply knowing what to expect, and how to deal with it.

For some people, coping with recovery symptoms is like riding a roller coaster. They will take sharp turns, slow climbs, and unexpected plunges. Most symptoms decrease after the first few days. Some stop totally after about three days. But some may get worse after a day or two. This may be partly psychological—the first day or two, your enthusiasm may keep you from recognizing some of your reactions to quitting. But most symptoms pass within two to four weeks.

Here are the most common symptoms, and the best ways to relieve them:

Symptom	Recommended Response
Irritability	Relaxercise, use the ideas about stress management in Step 6, take walks, hot baths, use nicotine replacement.
Fatigue	Take naps, try to take it easy—cut yourself some slack. Try nicotine replacement.
Insomnia	Relaxercise. Avoid caffeine, including , chocolate, after 6 P.M.
Cough, dry throat, nasal drip	Drink plenty of fluids, use cough drops.
Dizziness	Use extra caution driving, operating machinery, climbing stairs; change positions slowly.
Poor concentration	Plan workload accordingly. Avoid unnecessarily demanding assignments during the first week
Constipation, gas	Drink plenty of fluids, add roughage to diet (fruits, vegetables, whole grain cereals).
Hunger	Drink water or low-calorie liquids. Be prepared with low-calorie snacks.
Craving for a cigarette	Try Creative Alternatives, wait out the urge (urges last only a few minutes), distract yourself, exercise, go for a walk.

Don't Panic!

No matter how hard you plan, you're sure to hit a few situations where you're really dying for a cigarette. Don't panic!

QUICK QUIT TIP
The Four D's

Craving a cigarette is often the most difficult side effect of quitting. If you have trouble remembering all your Creative Alternatives, or if you're caught without a plan but with a really strong craving, think of the "four Ds":

1. **D**elay. The urge to smoke will pass whether you smoke or not.
2. **D**eep breathing (the essence of Relaxercise).
3. **D**rink water (drinking plenty of liquids helps ease many of the symptoms of quitting).
4. **D**o something to take your mind off smoking (check your Creative Alternatives).

And don't forget your list of alternative activities. Chew on a stirring stick. If you're using nicotine gum, remember to chew it frequently during the day. Doodle. Make a telephone call. Take a walk. Even if you're inside at home or in an office, you can walk into another room, pick up something to read for a few minutes, or go to the bathroom and brush your teeth.

QUICK QUIT TIP

REMEMBER: The urge to smoke will pass whether you smoke or not.

If you're still finding it hard to control the urge, call one of your key friends or family members. Follow through on your plan to contact with them for encouragement. If you need their help, even just to hear you rant and rave, don't be bashful. Remember, this is one of the most important and hardest things you'll do all year.

GET A PENCIL AND TRY THIS!

If you're feeling a bit strange today, without a cigarette in your hand, try this. Take out a blank piece of paper. Put a pen or pencil in your "wrong" hand (the hand you don't write with). Then put your other hand behind your back.

Now write your name and phone number on the piece of paper. How did it feel? Probably very awkward and difficult. Perhaps you felt silly or even incompetent. That's what happens anytime you do something new or that you are not used to. You think you don't do it well.

It's the same for quitting smoking. At first, you may feel different, awkward, uncomfortable, and inadequate. But it will become less difficult if you have good support and enough practice.

You've Planned Your Work, Now Work Your Plan

We all know that plans are easier to make than to keep. The American Lung Association's experience has shown us that people often stop doing the things that will help them stay off cigarettes. They may get distracted by their own discomfort or by other activities in their lives or they may just "forget," just as many of us forgot to practice for our music lessons when we were children or forgot our New Year's resolution by January 3rd!

Make sticking to your plan a priority. Here's where two of this book's main points come in.

1. Quitting smoking is one of the most important things you'll do all year. It deserves your time and attention even if that means putting some other important things "on hold" a little.
2. Healthy selfishness: If you slip or relapse, you will be responsible. But, it's your right, today and for the next few weeks and months, to do the things you need to do to stay off cigarettes.

Immediate Benefits

Right now, while you're concentrating on getting through the day without smoking, it's probably difficult to focus on the benefits of quitting. But this can be a great tool for success. For many people, recognizing benefits is an excellent source of motivation to keep on resisting the urge.

Did you know that your body is already starting to show the benefits of quitting? In fact, the moment you quit smoking, your body began to repair the damage. Within a half hour of your last cigarette, your blood pressure and pulse rate began to move back towards normal. Within merely eight hours, the carbon monoxide level in your blood dropped to normal and your oxygen level increased.

"JUSTIN"

Justin is quitting today. He knows it's not going to be easy. Yesterday his boss scheduled a meeting with a very powerful potential client, and Justin had to stay late to prepare for it. At the meeting, he knows he'll have to sit with his colleague, Henry, who's a pack-a-day smoker.

Rather than putting off his Quit Day, Justin surprised himself by taking the initiative to talk to Henry. He couldn't believe it when Henry offered to leave the meeting room for smoke breaks. Henry was happy to help his friend and, knowing the new client didn't smoke, Henry felt it was better not to risk offending the client by smoking in such an enclosed area.

Justin felt proud of how he had put a priority on his important personal goal. And he was very grateful to know that his old friend, Henry, was so willing to help him.

When he got up in the morning, Justin breezed through his one-mile run. He put on his favorite tie and left for work in a good mood. He felt confident that quitting smoking was going to work out all right.

**By quitting for just one day,
you have already decreased your chance
of having a sudden heart attack!**

You're well on the road to a longer, healthier, happier life. Congratulations! You're a nonsmoker now!

CHAPTER 10

Step 6
Your First Two
Nonsmoking Weeks

Congratulations! You've made it past your first day without smoking. You may not have thought you could do it . . . but you have! Think a little about how you feel about this. Many of us let our victories go almost unnoticed as we move ahead to the next crisis or item on our "to do" list. Why do you think you were successful? Where did you almost trip but keep going? How did you manage to avoid getting tripped up? How does this make you feel about your chances of staying off cigarettes? Somewhere in your answers to these questions, you may even feel a little proud of yourself!

You probably don't feel like a "new person yet," but you are already changing. You're likely to feel more energetic and more alive than you have in years. A lot of self-repair work is already going on inside you. Your body is at work repairing smoke-damaged tissues this very minute. You may not notice the changes yet, but you will.

It's a Tough Job

Reading about the wonderful advantages of quitting may not be so comforting to you if you're feeling symptoms of recovery. You may feel very cranky. You may have discovered nerves you never knew you had. You may be ready to take someone's head off for the silliest reason. You may even wish that you'd turn on the morning news and hear "Headline story—scientists have determined that smoking is not deadly after all."

All these feelings are normal, even if you're having them all at once. It's no secret that quitting smoking can be a very tough job. Remember that you have accomplished things successfully when you were angry. You've accomplished things when you were nervous, and you have accomplished things when you felt sick. Your physical and emotional feelings don't have to direct your actions. You can quit in spite of them!

QUICK QUIT TIP

WHEN WILL MY CRAVING FOR A CIGARETTE STOP?

The first week is usually the worst. After that, the cravings lessen and lessen. Each day you will feel better and better.

But be assured, *things will get better.* Most of these symptoms don't last long—a week or two at the most! Of course, right now a week or two seems like a long time. But remember, after your first week of not smoking, the nicotine finally will be out of your system, and much of the tension you feel, as well as some of the other physical symptoms, will disappear.

This isn't to say that you won't still have cravings after the first week. You probably will. But they'll become weaker and less frequent, and easier to deal with.

Learning anything new is tough at first. But it gets easier after the first few weeks.

Right now, though, you're still in the learning stage. Quitting is an extended process, not a single act. You still need help to learn to become a permanent non-smoker.

REFRAMING THE TASK

Would you like to enjoy life without smoking and without frequent urges for cigarettes? Here's a way you can accomplish this:

Go six months without a cigarette.

In my 20 years of helping people quit, not one person who'd gone six months without a cigarette ever said he or she wanted to go back to smoking. Most said they had thoughts about smoking but not real urges to smoke, and those who did have urges said they were not very frequent. Those who relapsed after this point usually were in a tight spot and made the mistake of thinking they could have just one. Those who have stayed off many years recognize they can't do that.

So think of yourself as working now to get where you want to be, enjoying life without missing cigarettes. Today's withdrawal symptoms and urges are not typical of what you have to look forward to. They will get better and your task of going six months without a cigarette will start getting easier after just a few more days—if not sooner.

Breaking the Nicotine Addiction Cycle

The *physical recovery* may be the most difficult during the first week or two. When you were smoking, you felt nervous and tense when your body craved nicotine. When you smoked a cigarette, you felt better because this craving was temporarily satisfied. But as the nicotine disappeared from your system, your nicotine craving again increased, and you again felt nervous and tense.

THE NICOTINE ADDICTION/STRESS CYCLE		
Drug induced Stress	*Drug induced Relief*	*Drug induced Stress*
I feel nervous and and tense because my body needs a cigarette.	I feel relaxed now that I have had a cigarette and I have temporarily satisfied my addiction.	I feel nervous and tense because my body needs a cigarette again.

You've quit smoking now, but your body is still caught up in the nicotine addiction stress cycle. You have withdrawn the addictive substance—nicotine—and that's caused a traumatic jolt to your whole body. The result for many people is a huge assortment of changes in your eating, sleeping, breathing, digestion, elimination, thinking, and everything else your body does.

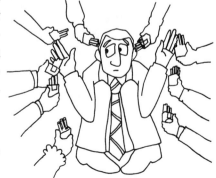

Learning anything new is tough at first. But it gets easier.

What's important to remember is that while you were taking nicotine by smoking many times each day, your body *wasn't* functioning normally. It seemed normal to you. But actually, you were continuously "under the influence" of nicotine. Now that the nicotine is gone, your body is working to relearn what is normal.

Signs of Physical Recovery

Right now, you are probably all too familiar with some of the symptoms of nicotine withdrawal. Reading about them won't make them go away. But understanding them may make them a little easier to tolerate. Most importantly, remember these are not new problems that have now become part of your life. They're just your body getting back to normal. We've mentioned this several times not because we want to preach about the virtue of being natural, but because it is helpful to keep this in mind.

Irritability is perhaps the most commonly reported reaction of people giving up cigarettes. In removing the effects of nicotine as well as hundreds of other chemicals found in smoke, you've caused your body considerable stress. It's understandable that you may feel short-fused for the first few days. Knowing to expect this normal reaction may help to keep it under control. Remember, cut yourself some slack and don't expect to be "perfect" during this stressful period.

Nervousness often accompanies irritability. You might want to ask your family, friends, and coworkers to try to understand that this is only a temporary effect that will disappear. Drink lots of liquids, especially fruit juices, to flush the nicotine out of your system as fast as possible. And avoid or limit stimulants like caffeine in coffee and cola drinks. Try the decaffeinated varieties.

Coughing may increase, too, because your lungs are cleaning themselves out, getting rid of residues built up from years of smoking. This "ex-smoker's cough" is temporary and usually lasts only a week or two at most. Cough drops or cough syrups should relieve it in the meantime.

A SURPRISING SYMPTOM—
INCREASED PRODUCTIVE COUGH

Smoking deadens the cilia in the lungs. These are little hairlike cells that help brush out dust and other residues in normal, healthy lungs. One of the reasons smokers have more infections is that their cilia are not working, so foreign matter accumulates in their lungs.

When you quit, the cilia get back to work within a couple of days. The result: you *start* coughing up *more* phlegm and sputum. Sometimes, ex-smokers get scared by this and think they have a new problem. But it's not that at all, just another example of your body getting back to normal.

Slight sore throat is also common. Although tobacco irritates your throat, it also numbs it. So when you stop smoking, you may feel some brief discomfort as your throat returns to its natural, normal state. Water and fruit juices can help.

Constipation is another frequent result of the body's readjusting to lack of nicotine. Drink plenty of water and supplement your diet with fiber from fruits and whole grains.

Sleeping problems result from tension. Use Relaxercise and other relaxation techniques. Exercise also helps work off nervous tension and helps you sleep better.

If you fall asleep normally, but wake in the middle of the night, you may be missing the nicotine your brain had gotten used to. Consider using a nicotine replacement product during the day to give your body some of the nicotine it's missing. If you still have trouble sleeping, talk to your doctor.

Tiredness often occurs as your body readjusts to functioning without the artificial stimulation of nicotine, especially if you're having trouble sleeping. You may have headaches, too. Try to increase your exercise or allow yourself a little extra time for sleeping.

Difficulty concentrating can be another consequence of

quitting. Many smokers have learned to rely on nicotine for alertness. In a short time, you will find this gets better. Your intense focus on quitting may also cause your mind to block out other thoughts. Nicotine replacement therapy can help here, too.

The Psychological Recovery Process

Many smokers are only slightly bothered by physical symptoms of nicotine withdrawal, but experience a lot more trouble with the psychological symptoms of recovery. Getting over the psychological loss can be very complex. It may even take several months for you to restructure a lifestyle without smoking.

Our reaction to giving up smoking can be like our reaction to death. Something dear to you is gone forever. It was something that was dangerous, but it was something that you were used to and liked in many ways, maybe because it made you feel sophisticated or able to handle things or attractive or sexy. Maybe it relaxed you and put you in a better mood.

Think of giving up smoking like the death of a close friend. Cigarettes have been your friend. They were always there for you. They didn't tell you that you were making mistakes or that you were being unreasonable. They never got angry at you or demanding (except when you ran out in the middle of the night). Instead, they made you feel more relaxed and confident about what you were doing.

Almost anytime we experience a major change in our life, we grieve for the old order before we can make room for the new. In her research on adjusting to the prospect of death, Elisabeth Kübler-Ross identified five stages in the grieving process in her book *Death and Dying*:

1. Denial
2. Anger
3. Depression
4. Bargaining
5. Acceptance

Let's look at how this relates to quitting smoking.

Denial is our mind's first way of protecting us from a sudden change or loss. People who lose a friend or family member say they feel numb. This is what we call a psychological defense mechanism. All mentally healthy people have this defense. For a smoker, this means that, although you know the importance of quitting, you may not want to believe it. Here are some common denial statements:

- ▶ "I know I should quit, but I'm not sure I want to."
- ▶ "Cigarettes don't affect my health like they do others. I'm not huffing and puffing."
- ▶ "Cigarettes haven't been proven harmful."
- ▶ "I'm not addicted."
- ▶ "This quitting thing is easy—I can do it anytime, just not today."

You've already started the quitting process, so you've gone past this denial stage. Or have you? Have you found yourself thinking things like:

- ▶ "If I'm having trouble quitting, it wouldn't be so terrible to go back to smoking."
- ▶ "Hey, it's just not a good time for me. I can do this again . . ."
- ▶ "I'm young. By the time I get old enough to get lung cancer, they'll have a cure."
- ▶ "I keep my weight down and I use seatbelts and I don't drink too much, so one 'vice' isn't going to do me in."

These are attempts to deny the problem rather than deal with it. We all do it. But you don't want to be talked into a mistake by this human tendency.

Anger often surfaces when we begin to accept a loss. Most smokers are angry about having to make a change in their lives. They feel their "friend" was taken away unfairly. They're angry because they feel singled out. Some typical angry thoughts people have may be:

- ▶ "Why me? I'm mad I started and mad I had to quit."
- ▶ "Why didn't someone tell us cigarettes are so harmful?"
- ▶ "Lucky nonsmokers. They have it easy."
- ▶ "Why does it have to be so hard to quit?"
- ▶ "What about people who are overweight? I don't see everyone getting on their case."

Notice that each of the statements of resentment contains a

sense of having been hurt, treated unfairly, or forced to do something really hard but without others helping very much. All of these feelings are understandable. Smokers do have a tough job that others don't have. Nobody is able to give them as much help as they might want—others don't have the ability to fix it for you. It may be hard to admit, but if you can acknowledge feeling hurt and recognize that your hurt is justified, you'll be easier on yourself. And talking with your friends or family about feeling bad about giving up smoking, rather than biting their heads off, is likely to get you more useful encouragement.

Depression and sadness often occur when we accept the loss of our "friend." This is especially true when no one else seems to know our loss. People often experience this in one of two ways:

1. A deep sense of sadness, or
2. A deep sense of deprivation

You'll realize you're in the depression stage if you're thinking:

- ▶ "I feel so emotional."
- ▶ "I feel so deprived."
- ▶ "Why can't I have this one little habit?"
- ▶ "Life without cigarettes is awful."
- ▶ "I feel so lonely."

Some might call this the "ain't it awful" stage. You feel as though you've lost a good friend. Well, you have. As with any loss, you need to take this in. Then, when you move on, you can recognize what holes you have to fill, needs you have to meet in new ways. Don't resist this stage or think it's crazy to mourn the loss of a cigarette. Take some time and give yourself the right just to feel sad.

Bargaining is the stage where smokers want to postpone the inevitable. You want to do all sorts of good things in return for a little lightening of the load of giving up cigarettes. You may try making deals with yourself like:

- ▶ "I think I have the worst licked. If I have just one cigarette, I'll get right back on track afterward and I won't do it again."
- ▶ "I'll quit for a week and then reward myself by smoking only on weekends."
- ▶ "I'll quit as long as my weight stays down. But if it goes up, I'll have to choose. Better to smoke and not gain weight."

Everyone is tempted to bargain. Realizing that it is a natural part of the process of quitting sometimes helps you to move past it. Laugh it off and have a heart-to-heart talk with the "child" inside you.

But you do need to stay on your toes with bargaining. When you really *want* a cigarette, that bargain can seem *very* reasonable. You may want to make a promise with one of your friends or family members that you will talk it over with them before you follow any plan that includes smoking some cigarettes. They may be able to help you see through the bargain that is about to interrupt your campaign.

Acceptance is the stage at which you begin to realize your former smoking lifestyle is over. You are finally resolving your sense of loss or grief. A healthy person who has suffered a loss eventually accepts its reality and goes on living life. Some typical comments of acceptance are:

> ► "I think I'm going to do this. I still don't like it a lot, but I think it will stick. "
> ► "I'd still like to smoke sometimes, but I choose not to."
> ► "I am going to teach myself to like my new nonsmoking lifestyle. I'll do it gradually and positively."

With acceptance, you combine all the stages that came before. You don't deny that quitting is hard, but you do find your mind moving on to other things. You stop being angry, but you remain annoyed that the tobacco companies suckered you into hurting yourself. You don't make a bargain of two weeks of good deeds in exchange for a cigarette, but you do recognize now that cigarettes are no longer a source of satisfaction in your life, and that you need and deserve to find other things that make you feel happy and relaxed.

You can get on with living your newfound, healthier lifestyle. A key to moving through these stages to psychological recovery is your attitude toward them. Look at them as part of

You're in charge of your own life again. You have regained your sense of self-control.

the process. Don't be thrown or surprised by them. You may even be able to work up a sense of challenge, expectation, and excitement over what lies ahead for you.

SOME PERSPECTIVES TO HELP YOU THROUGH

▶ Reject the feeling that you have given something up. It's quite the opposite—you have gained something—your freedom and self-mastery.

▶ This is not an exercise in self-denial, but self-determination. You're now in charge of your life again. You have a tremendous sense of self-control.

▶ You are giving a gift to yourself and to those near you.

▶ You're getting rid of a harmful habit. You're working hard, and you're getting important benefits in return.

▶ You deserve a lot of praise for your efforts. Give yourself a big pat on the back. Reward yourself in small and big ways.

Replacing the Psychological Benefits of Cigarettes

As you go through the stages of physical and psychological recovery, you will have lots of feelings. Chewing stirring sticks or going for walks might help control urges to smoke when you're bored or fidgety. But these Creative Alternatives won't do as long-term substitutes for the cigarettes you use to control your feelings.

WAS *THAT* WHAT I WAS REALLY FEELING WHEN I SMOKED?

A wise friend once pointed out that almost every time she lit a cigarette, she realized she was *not* saying something that she felt. When you're on the spot, lighting up gives you a few seconds to collect your thoughts. When you're hurt or annoyed, giving yourself a cigarette can help you overlook the fact that you're unhappy and put up with whatever is bothering you. Of course, the nicotine improves your mood too, so smoking becomes both a psychological and chemical way of covering your feelings.

As you get used to life without nicotine, you'll rediscover some of the feelings that smoking supressed.

Not smoking will be easier if you keep in touch with your feelings, likes, dislikes, worries, and irritations. Start taking your feelings into account. Instead of just saying to yourself, "I need a cigarette," ask yourself what feeling is leading you to this. If you can get in touch with that feeling, you can begin to find better ways than smoking to handle it.

When tempted to reach for a cigarette, ask:

▶ What am I feeling?

▶ Why am I having this feeling?

▶ What do I really want now?

Usually what you want is *not* a cigarette. Here are two examples:

▶ Tom walked into a big party knowing no one. He immediately felt uncomfortable. His eyes scanned the room looking for a friendly face, but everyone seemed deeply involved in conversation with someone else. Tom felt conspicuous standing there doing nothing. Boy, did he want a cigarette.

▶ Rita was eating lunch with her coworkers. Everyone else was discussing their children. Since Rita had no children, she was not interested in the topic. Feeling excluded, she noticed how much she missed a cigarette after lunch.

Instead of wanting cigarettes, what Tom and Rita want is to feel included. Luckily there are other responses that will address this. Tom could offer to help the host serve drinks as a way of comfortably starting to talk with other guests. He could gather up his courage and approach someone else who is standing alone, and start a conversation. Rita could join another group for lunch, or think about how she is curious about what it's like to have kids and ask questions about it.

Chapter 13 has some specific ways of learning to deal with the feelings that may cause you to want a cigarette. If you find yourself having urges to smoke when you are feeling shy or uncomfortable, stressed, or stuck with family or relationship conflicts, try to find new ways to deal with those feelings.

Alternatives for Handling Bad Moods

Sometimes you feel sad, anxious, or frustrated for good reasons. Bad things do happen. But there are other times you may get down on yourself because you're judging yourself too harshly or negatively. If you're like most people, you sometimes blow things out of proportion or over-react to incidents you'd generally find

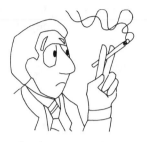

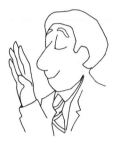

Smokers who don't succeed in quitting think:: cigarettes do a lot for me— they're always there for me.

Smokers who quit shift to: cigarettes deprive me of life and health.

only mildly annoying. And, as much as it happens to all of us, blowing things out of proportion can be a big problem when you're quitting smoking.

Once you quit smoking, what else can you do? Here are a few practical alternatives:

▶ **Check your assumptions.** When you're upset or in a bad mood, write down what you're thinking and feeling. Then question why you feel the way you do. For example, suppose you feel depressed because your coworkers forgot your birthday. That is upsetting, but does it really mean they don't care about you? If you feel loved by your family and you have your fair share of good friends, does it really matter if your coworkers didn't remember your special occasion?

CHECK YOUR ASSUMPTIONS

Here are some assumptions you may be making about yourself. They may make you feel badly about yourself and may make you want to smoke:

1. I should never disappoint anyone.
2. I need to be loved or liked by everyone.
3. I should be such a good and worthy person that everyone will treat me with respect.
4. In order to be happy, I have to be successful in everything I do.
5. If I make a mistake, it shows I'm not really very good.
6. If someone disagrees with me, it means they don't like me or don't think much of me.

7. My worth as a person depends on what other people—every one of them—think of me.

8. Life is fair. If I am a nice person, if I'm cheerful, if I do my best for others, bad things won't happen to me. If bad things do happen to me, it means I just haven't been good enough.

▶ **Change your expectations.** If you find yourself expecting to be perfect with your family, if you find yourself feeling you always need to be on time, if you find yourself upset whenever anyone shows they're less than delighted with you—whatever may be the mistakes you're making in judging yourself—try to figure out a more realistic way of looking at things. Suppose needing always to be perfect is your downfall. Try thinking of a better way of looking at things. You might think about a friend who isn't perfect but seems to do a lot of good things and enjoy life. Practice thinking about this person when you're tempted to expect too much of yourself. Work on it ahead of time, so you'll have it when you need it.

CHANGING HOW YOU THINK ABOUT YOURSELF

Here are some approaches to combating the assumptions that make you feel bad:

1. Pretend you are your best friend. How would you argue with the assumptions you are making? What would your best friend tell you to help you feel better about yourself?

2. Think about how much you might enjoy life if you didn't carry around the assumptions that are making you feel bad.
   - What would it be like if you only wanted to be *competent*, not perfect?
   - What would it be like if you were content to feel that *half of your coworkers* were your friends and didn't need to feel you had to be friends with all of them?
   - What would it be like if you were satisfied that your children know *you love them* and that you do your best even if you sometimes do make mistakes?

3. Work out a logical argument—pretend you're a lawyer—against the way you're looking at yourself. Practice the argument so you'll be able to recall it when you're tempted to blow things out of proportion.

4. Write down some things to remind yourself when you're tempted to feel bad. Carry the list with you so you can look at it when you're in the sort of situation that tends to make you upset.

5. As suggested earlier, imagine a friend who does a good job of handling the situations that upset you. Imagine what positive thoughts they may have about themselves in these situations. Now think of yourself being positive in the same way. Practice this and remember it when you get into upsetting situations.

The Reward Cigarette

We've been talking about how stress and bad feelings can lead to cravings. But many people also smoke when they feel good. If you're one of them, you may often think, "I deserve this cigarette!"

After you've quit smoking, you won't be able to reward yourself with a cigarette. So you'll have to work on new rewards:

▶ Ask yourself what healthy activity would make you feel good right now, would make you feel rewarded.

▶ Make a list-do this ahead of time—of nonsmoking activities to do to make yourself feel good: call a good friend long distance, go to a movie, etc.

Positive Self-Talk

Positive Self-Talk—telling yourself good things about yourself—can be a good way to combat bad moods. Many people spend too much time telling themselves they can't do things, aren't doing a good job, aren't capable. That's *negative* Self-Talk. Positive Self-Talk simply reverses all that, by changing the negative thoughts into "I can do it" statements.

Consider this situation: A coworker asks you to join her, as usual, for a coffee break, which always includes smoking.

You could think, and tell yourself, the following negative Self-Talk:

▶ I'll never be able to stick this out and say "no" to a cigarette.

▶ I really love sitting at the table with a cigarette and coffee at breaktime.

▶ I don't want to hurt her feelings by not smoking with her.

Or, you could try some Positive Self-Talk:

▶ I can do it if I take one day at a time. It will get easier with time if I just persist.

▶ I can get the same relaxed feeling if I sit and chat with a cup of tea and the crossword puzzle

▶ I feel good when I do what's *really* good for me. This decision to quit smoking is important to me.

So, which one would you choose? Obviously the Positive Self-Talk will do better to help you cope with strong urges, as well as help you develop attitudes and self-perceptions that are important in becoming a successful long-term nonsmoker.

POSITIVE SELF-STATEMENTS

When stress starts to escalate, use any of these positive self-statements to help you think more rationally and calmly.

1. I should think about what I *really* want for myself.
2. Relax. I can calm down with a slow, deep breath.
3. I can handle this. Take one step at a time.
4. This is a chance for me to use what I have learned.
5. Tough times don't last.
6. Look for solutions.
7. Stop. Look on the positive side.
8. I can get support, advice, and help if I need it.

MORE ON PERSPECTIVES

Smokers who don't succeed in quitting have his attitude:	*Smokers who quit shift to this:*
▶ Cigarettes do a lot for me. They're kind of like a friend. They're always there when I when I need them.	▶ Cigarettes make me cough, feel breathless,trigger heart trouble, and cause lung cancer.
▶ Quitting deprives me.	▶ Cigarettes deprive me—of life and health.
▶ I resent feeling deprived.	▶ Quitting has shown me personal strengths I didn't know I had.

Visualization

Visualization is another positive technique. Take a few moments every day to close your eyes and visualize yourself as a non-smoker. "See" yourself *not smoking* in many situations—at work, at home, in social situations, or out at restaurants. When you're doing your Relaxercises, begin to visualize yourself as a healthy person with clean lungs. In fact, you're not just visualizing that—it's actually happening!

You can also use visualization to rehearse some of your Do Power strategies. If you have a specific plan for handling a key temptation, visualize yourself carrying it through and succeeding in staying on the path to your goal.

Managing Stress

Facing down your smoking triggers without smoking isn't easy. It's often quite stressful. Physical cravings for nicotine also cause stress. When you were a smoker, you usually used cigarettes to reduce your stress. Now you seem to have no skills for dealing with stressful situations.

You need both short-term and long-term solutions to stress. The short-term help will get you through the day. The long-term solution is to figure out what's causing the stress and try to change it. Step 7 has some long-term solutions to stressors. If stress is a big factor in your urge to smoke, check it out.

Exercise is a great way to combat stress. Tactics to reduce stress are like Do Power—what is great for one person may sound silly to another. Here are some to consider:

STRESS REDUCERS

1. Get up 15 minutes earlier in the morning. The inevitable morning mishaps will be less stressful.

2. Prepare for the morning the evening before. Set the breakfast table. Make lunches. Put out the clothes you plan to wear.

3. Don't rely on your memory. Write down appointment times, when to pick up the laundry, when library books are due, etc.

4. Make copies of all keys. Bury a house key in a secret spot in the garden. Carry a duplicate car key in your wallet.

5. Practice preventive maintenance. Your car, appliances, home, and relationships will be less likely to break down at the "worst possible moment."

6. Be prepared to wait. A paperback book can make a wait in line almost pleasant.

7. Procrastination is stressful. Whatever you want to do tomorrow, do today. Whatever you want to do today, do it now.

8. Plan ahead. Don't let the gas tank get below one-quarter full. Keep a well-stocked "emergency shelf" of home staples. Don't wait until you're down to your last bus token or postage stamp to buy more.

9. Don't put up with something that doesn't work right. If your alarm clock, wallet, shoe laces—whatever—are a constant aggravation, fix them or get new ones.

10. Allow 15 minutes extra time to get to appointments. Plan to arrive at an airport one hour before your flight.

11. Eliminate (or restrict) the caffeine in your diet.

12. Relax your standards. The world will not end if the grass doesn't get mowed this weekend.

13. Pollyanna-Power! For every one thing that goes wrong, there are probably 10 or 50 or one hundred blessings.

14. Say "No!" Saying no to extra projects, social activities, and invitations you know you don't have the time or energy for takes practice, self-respect, and a belief that everyone, needs quiet time to relax and to be alone. Unplug your phone when you want to take a long bath, meditate, sleep, or read without interruption.

Relaxercise can be a great way to cope with stress. In most instances, this quick relaxation exercise can help a craving to pass. As an ex-smoker, you may have another reason to focus on deep-breathing relaxation. When you smoked, you often inhaled deeply in a way that actually promoted relaxation. People who stop smoking often forget to continue such deep breathing, and so they experience increased tension.

Deep Breathing Techniques

This exercise will show you how to breathe without cigarettes in a way that slows down the pace of your whole body and, therefore, promotes general relaxation. Deep breathing should be done using your stomach muscles as well as your lungs.

Before doing the exercise, put a hand on your abdomen. As you inhale deeply, feel your stomach pull in toward your spine. When you exhale, feel your stomach muscles release. As you do the exercise, pause comfortably at the end of each exhalation until you feel ready to take the next deep breath.

It may be helpful to think of your lungs as balloons that you are trying to fill as completely as possible.

1. Breathe in deeply, letting your stomach expand until your lungs are filled. Pause for a moment and then exhale until you have emptied your lungs.

2. Pause for a moment, then take another deep breath in, filling your lungs from the bottom.

3. Hold for a moment . . . and now let the airflow out, focusing your mind on restful thoughts.

4. Keeping the pace regular, again breathe in deeply . . . hold a moment . . . and now let the air out, feeling more and more relaxed.

5. Take another breath in . . . hold it for a moment . . . now gently breathe out, letting the tension escape from your body.

6. Once more breathe in . . . pause a moment .. . now exhale, feeling deep relaxation.

SOMEONE WHO REALLY LEARNED HOW TO TAKE A POSITIVE VIEW: "I quit smoking three times before this time. I know the difference between this time and the others. The first three times, I always felt deprived. This time I changed my thinking. I admitted I was only deprived of the burns, the stink, and all the negatives about smoking. I admitted that I was controlled by the cigarette. Then I decided I would take back my control. I became determined instead of deprived."—Katie, age 39

After you've learned how to do it, you can achieve even greater relaxation if you close your eyes during deep breathing. Let your mind focus on a restful scene or a word like "calm" to give you a feeling of mental quiet.

New Do Power Strategies

Now that you're a nonsmoker, you need to review your Do Power plans for coping with temptations (see Chapter 3, page 47). Look back at the temptations you identified in Step 4 and the plans you had for coping with them. Which ones have you tried so far? Which ones have worked and which ones haven't worked as well as you expected?

Based on your results so far, you may want to revise your list. Use the following work sheet to identify things you have done that did help you stay away from cigarettes. Now think of two or three situations coming up this week that may make you want to smoke. Then write in things you could do instead of smoking.

You may also want to treat moods and feelings like temptations. Just as you may have a Do Power strategy for the temptation of morning coffee, you can develop a Do Power strategy for emotions that will make you want to smoke. For example, if you can *antici-pate* that a deadline next Monday is going to make you anxious over the weekend, try to identify some *specific* things you can *do* to keep yourself from smoking. You might:

▶ Take extra care to allow yourself ample time for the task, so meeting your deadline won't be so stressful.

▶ Plan fifteen-minute walks both morning and afternoon over the weekend to keep things a little calmer.

▶ Ask your spouse to give you encouragement over the weekend. Be sure to say exactly how you want to be encouraged—a pep talk or a hug, for example.

▶ Plan your work so you can take a 10 minute Relaxercise break every hour.

▶ Make sure you plan some things you'll enjoy doing over the weekend so the anxiety of making the deadline won't be compounded by feeling sad that you don't have enough fun.

▶ Make sure the area where you work doesn't have any reminders of smoking so you are not caught off guard.

None of these may be the right Do Power strategy for you. Identify your specific temptations and come up with specific strategies that you feel good about.

QUICK QUIT TIP:

Drinking alcohol will increase your urge to smoke.

"For the first few weeks after quitting, I held myself to just a drink or two at the most. Any more than that just gave me a real urge to smoke."—Stephen, age 41

Remember, quitting smoking is a long process. You must continue to work on your Do Power. People lapse when they let temptations come over them without doing anything about them. It doesn't matter so much what you do as long as it makes sense for you. But you do need to do something to keep those temptations at bay.

NEW DO POWER STRATEGIES

**List two temptations and, for each,
two Do Power strategies you have used successfully
in the past.**

Situation   *Do Power Strategy*

1. _____   _____

2. _____   _____

**Now name two situations coming up this week that may
make you want to smoke. Then write in things you could
do instead of smoking.**

Situation   *Do Power Strategy*

Example: Drinks with   ▶ Don't go this time.
friends after work.   ▶ Go, but drink club soda.

1. _____   _____

2. _____   _____

**Now write down a feeling that will make you
want to smoke and some Do Power strategies
for coping with it.**

Situation   *Do Power Strategy*

Example: Sad or blue.   ▶ Go to a movie.
                ▶ Make phone calls to old
                   friends.

1. _____   _____

2. _____   _____

What If Do Power Doesn't Work

Nobody's perfect. There will be times when all your Creative Alternatives and Do Power don't keep a temptation from being a tough one. When things don't go well, ask yourself:

- ▶ Could I have anticipated the temptation sooner?
- ▶ Did I look at all aspects of the temptation situation that I could change or avoid?
- ▶ Did I make a concrete plan?
- ▶ Did I carry out my plan or just think about it?

Different control strategies work for different people. Don't give up if a strategy that works for other people fails for you. Try something else! Persevere and be creative. You *can* find a strategy to avoid temptation.

Review the Do Power basics of specifying the temptation, being creative about thinking of strategies, and carrying out your plan. When you find that a little creativity and effort can help solve a temptation, you're going to be much happier!

> "I try to do deep breathing exercises, which I can—now that I can breathe. But when the stress gets really bad at work, I usually try to get up and you know, just walk around the room or walk around the office, or just bend over and touch my toes, or stretch, to just relieve the tension in the muscles."
> —Carlos, age 32

Really Tempted

By the time you're reading this section, you may have been smoke-free for five days, seven days, ten days, or even longer. Congratulations! You're doing a great job. And you're probably feeling more and more confident about being a nonsmoker.

But there have probably been several times when you've been tempted to "have just one." When the temptation is high, you may even think to yourself, "If I have just one cigarette, it's no big deal."

Don't kid yourself! Even one cigarette can hurt. One can lead to two. Two can lead to three. And before too long, you're liable to be back to buying cartons.

> ### QUICK QUIT TIP
> ## THE QUITTER'S PARADOX
>
> Having even one cigarette reduces your chances of success. You need to be determined that you will not smoke, not at all, not even a puff.
>
> Most successful quitters, however, have failed a few times before they got it right. For many, relapsing and trying again is part of learning to be a nonsmoker, sort of like skinning your knees is part of learning to ride a bicycle.
>
> *So* be as determined as you can be. Don't start letting yourself have a cigarette here, a cigarette there. *But*, if you do have a setback, don't get down on yourself. You are still on your way toward eventually being a nonsmoker.

What Happens If I Slip Up?

It's not the end of the world. Many people slip up and have a cigarette once or twice, but quickly get back on track. So if you do slip, it doesn't mean you've failed. If you get down on yourself, you aren't giving yourself a chance. So, give yourself a break: forgive yourself.

> ### QUICK QUIT TIP:
> ### If you get down on yourself,
> ### you aren't giving yourself a chance.
>
> **Wrong:** "I was good for two days and then I blew it! I'm ready to forget the whole thing."
> **Right:** "Quitting is a process and backsliding is just a part of it. If I can learn what went wrong this time, I'll do better next time."

Millions of people who have quit smoking slip and smoke. And many of these smokers still end up quitting. Here are some steps you can take to combat your slip-up:

- ▶ Stop smoking immediately.
- ▶ Take action. Throw away the cigarettes or leave the place where you smoked. Treat your situation like an emergency and get out of it.

Once you've removed yourself from the situation, look back and consider what went wrong. Where were you? What were you doing? Who were you with? Was it your mood that made you vulnerable?

▶ Analyze the situation, and learnwhat caused the slip.

▶ Prepare yourself for the next time. Ask yourself what you'll do if this situation happens again.

▶ If the problem was a temptation that got the best of you, review the Do Power tips above and in Step 4. Come up with a specific plan to combat the temptation next time.

If you have been using nicotine replacement therapy, take time now to review the package instructions. Perhaps you need an increase in your dosage or suggestions on how to use these products more effectively. If you're unsure, you might contact your doctor or pharmacist for instructions.

Your Inner Culprit

Of course, it's not always easy to get out of a slip-up. Even one slip can plunge people into a sense of helplessness and a feeling that failure is inevitable.

The reason this happens is that there's a part of you—your "inner culprit"—that would be relieved by proof that your case is hopeless, that the lapse proves it. Then you could just relax, recognize that "we all gotta go somehow," and simply accept your smoking and enjoy life.

People know this isn't really true. We all do "gotta go somehow," but smoking—more than anything else we do to ourselves—does a lot to make that day come sooner. That's why this book includes that chapter with all the depressing facts about how much damage smoking does. You may want to review it now if you find yourself wondering whether it really is worth it to stick this out. Of course, review your Top 5 Reasons for Not Smoking to keep clear on your own personal reasons for putting yourself through this.

Don't let the "inner culprit" give you justification for succumbing to temptation. There are two keys to fighting it:

▶ Recognize that quitting smoking is much more important than most of the other things you do for your health

▶ Remember that most ex-smokers relapsed several times before they succeeded, so you're just kidding yourself if you think your case is impossible

If you feel unsteady, go back to the Quitter's Checklist at the beginning of this Step. Figure out which things may be worth a little more time and effort.

Blockbusters to the Rescue!

Remember the six Blockbusters you read about in Chapter 3? We've already talked about Do Power but review the other Blockbusters now to see if you're using them as much as you might.

Blockbuster #1: Exercise. Have you been getting enough exercise? Remember, even a short walk can help you relax and give you something to do instead of smoking.

Blockbuster #2: Battling the bulges. If you're feeling discouraged because you've gained a few pounds, keep reminding yourself that those pounds aren't nearly as bad for you as smoking. Right now, your first priority is to stay off cigarettes. Later on, you can give more attention to your weight. But to prevent too many extra pounds from finding their way to your midsection, remember to stock up on smart snacks like fruits, fresh vegetables, popcorn, and dry cereal. Or keep a stirring stick around so you'll have something to put in your mouth and to occupy your hands.

Blockbuster #3: Assertive Responses. Did you almost have a cigarette because someone offered it to you? If so, now's the time to practice your Assertive Responses. What can you say the next time someone lights up and holds out the cigarette package to offer you one? A positive, direct, but nonaggressive response ("No thanks! I really do want to stay off cigarettes this time") can help you stay focused on your own priorities.

Were you tempted to smoke because you were upset about something somebody said and you didn't know what to say back?

You don't have to convince the other person or win the argument, but if you clearly state your own feelings, you'll feel a lot more true to yourself and less stirred up and needing a smoke.

> ***Blockbuster #4:*** Creative Alternatives. Are you especially tempted to smoke when you're feeling bored, stressed, or unhappy? Perhaps you've forgotten your list of Creative Alternatives to smoking. If you're bored, you could take a walk, doodle, work on a hobby, or call a friend. If you're stressed, you could Relaxercise, hit a pillow, do aerobics, or even yell and scream (in private, of course!). Review your own lists again.

> ***Blockbuster #5:*** Relaxercise. Are you remembering to Relaxercise at least once a day? If you're having difficulty staying quit, consider taking mini breaks throughout the day to Relaxercise. And whenever you're in a situation that tempts you to smoke, stop and Relaxercise. If that's not enough, find a quiet spot and do your Deep Breathing exercise (see page 144). *Remember, the urge will pass whether you smoke or not!*

> ***Blockbuster #6:*** Do Power. We've talked about this a lot in this step. Review your list of smoking triggers—and your alternatives to smoking in response to these triggers. Make sure you have the strategies to keep temptations from getting in the way of your goals.

Don't Go Down in Flames Alone

Remember your plans to get encouragement and cooperation from your friends and family. There's a tendency to think you have to do it alone. And if you find yourself stumbling, you may be even more reluctant to call on others for help. Remember that quitting smoking is important and that you have the right to expect cooperation from those around you. Call on your friends and family. They'll probably be flattered that you asked them for a little boost and be happy to cheer you on or assist your good efforts.

For additional encouragement, look around to find a few people who have quit smoking for more than a year. Ask them if they regret it!

Reviewing Your Progress

It's not easy to break a long-term habit like smoking. But you're doing it! If you've reached this point, you're motivated and determined. But the battle's not won yet. You'll have to stay vigilant.

One way to do this is to monitor your progress every day. Use the Progress Report below (make copies to use each day). Record the difficult situations you faced that day, and the coping techniques you used successfully. Then make a list of things you will do during the next day, instead of smoking.

PROGRESS REPORT

List the situations you ran into today that brought on strong urges to smoke. Then write down the coping techniques you successfully used to handle each of the situations.

Situations	*Do Power or other techniques I used successfully*
1. _____	1. _____
2. _____	2. _____
3. _____	3. _____
4. _____	4. _____

What I will do tomorrow instead of smoking:

(Some suggestions)   *Now think of your own:*

► Go to a double feature.   _____

► Take a long walk.   _____

► Visit a museum.   _____

► Practice deep breathing.   _____

► Sit in the nonsmoking
  lunchroom.   _____

►Spend time window-shopping. _____

"MARIA"

Things are going pretty well for Maria. She and Bruce are enjoying their evening walks together. She has two more sessions to go in her Freedom from Smoking group, and she's getting to be a real nut about those relaxation exercises—mostly because she enjoys them as something she does for herself every day.

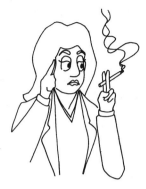

Two nights ago, it was raining, so she and Bruce couldn't take their usual walk. About an hour after dinner, she smelled cigarette smoke. Her first impulse was to feel angry and hurt that Bruce would tempt her this way. Then she realized that maybe he just didn't understand. She went into the

Ask yourself, "Why am I smoking this cigarette?

living room where he was watching TV and very calmly asked him if he'd do her a favor and put his cigarette out. When Bruce realized she wasn't angry with him, but was just asking for his help, he snuffed the cigarette out right away.

Then they worked out a compromise. They needed milk for breakfast, so Bruce took his cigarettes along and was able to smoke in the car on his way to the supermarket. He also brought home some chocolate fudge ice cream. Maria was delighted—although she did limit herself to a small serving. She has gained a few pounds since she stopped smoking and doesn't want it to get any worse than that. But it made her happy to know she could strike a good compromise—enjoying a little bit of ice cream, feeling good about not smoking, and appreciating Bruce's willingness to cooperate with her on some pretty difficult problems.

If you decided to sign a *Freedom From Smoking®* contract on your Quit Day, now's a good time to review it and maybe make another one with some dates for rewards in the month ahead. (see page 117) Enjoy thinking of some good rewards you can give yourself

"I went back to smoking when my friend at work offered me a cigarette. I hadn't told him that I had quit. I just took the cigarette. I learned my lesson! I've now told everyone I work with that I've quit for good. They don't offer me cigarettes anymore."—Richard, age 51

> "Every day I would get up in the morning and I would go to the mirror in the bathroom and I'd recite my reasons for wanting to quit out loud to myself. I felt somehow that it worked, that it made them more real to me. When I'd have an urge to smoke, I'd get out that list of reasons—I had it on a little index card. I'd recite the reasons out loud and somehow that helped to keep me off smoking."—Linda, age 25

for each week and each month you go without smoking.

If this seems repetitive, remember that relapses can occur for several months after quitting. Those old associations between cigarettes and all the times you used to smoke have not all gone away. Just as with all the other hard and important things you've done in your life, you need to give this one the attention it deserves until you've really got it licked.

But not all is toil and trouble. Each day you go without smoking puts you another day closer to becoming a confirmed nonsmoker—for life. That will take about six months. But think of something that happened six months ago. Seems like only yesterday, right? So this too shall pass, it will get easier, and you will get through the next weeks and months to arrive at your goal, nonsmoking and not missing 'em!

CHAPTER 11

Step 7
The First Six Months

You did it! You've quit smoking and stayed quit for two weeks.

That's great. You weren't sure you could do it, but you were able to. Not only a great boost for your health, but also for your pride!

Remember that the best way to get to the point where you enjoy life without missing cigarettes is by not smoking for six months. Step 7 is designed to get you there. Although "you've come a long way," you need to keep on your toes. In fact, one of the first things we talk about below is not relaxing too soon because you feel so successful.

QUITTER'S CHECKLIST

Put a check in the space next to each strategy or technique you have worked on. If there are a lot of empty spaces, you may want to increase your effort here.

- ❑ Top 5 Reasons for Not Smoking
- ❑ Do Power
- ❑ Relaxercise
- ❑ Creative Alternatives
- ❑ Blockbuster #1 Exercise
- ❑ Blockbuster #2: Battling the bulges
- ❑ Blockbuster #3: Assertive responses
- ❑ Getting cooperation and encouragement from family and friends
- ❑ Planning and giving yourself rewards for progress

New in Step 6:
- ❑ Working on psychological recovery—getting through Bargaining and Depression to get to Acceptance
- ❑ Replacing psychological benefits of cigarettes—finding other ways to cope with anxiety or sadness
- ❑ Checking your assumptions and expectations to avoid or stop bad moods
- ❑ Replacing the Reward Cigarette—finding other ways to reward yourself
- ❑ Using Positive Self Talk
- ❑ Practicing Visualization
- ❑ Managing stress
- ❑ Using Deep Breathing
- ❑ Remembering the Quitter's Paradox: Be determined but don't be discouraged if you slip
- ❑ Fighting the "inner culprit"—don't think your case is hopeless if you slip

Don't Let Success Cause You to Fail

At this point you may feel quitting has been easier than you expected. Not that it's been easy altogether, but it still has not been as hard as you feared. You may now go for several hours, maybe most of the day or evening, without even thinking about a cigarette.

Here's the downside of feeling too confident: You're at a party. You're feeling good. Maybe you've had a drink or two. Someone offers you a cigarette. You think, "I'm not having any trouble. I'll have a couple tonight and go back to non-smoking tomorrow. Maybe stay with a routine of only smoking at parties."

> You want to develop the habit of not smoking, until it becomes just that. A habit. Something you don't think about. Something you just do.

One of the first times I quit, I decided I'd only smoke on weekends. Soon, I was trying to convince myself that the weekend begins on Wednesday evening and ends the following Wednesday morning!

Vigilance—that's the word for the next few months. You

don't have to spend every waking moment managing your quitting, but you do have to stay on your toes, vigilant, alert to the temptations or situations that can mess up your plan. Give your nonsmoking the vigilance you would for anything else that is very important.

If You Slip ...

If you have one or two slips, go back to the Step 6 directions for handling slips. If you've gone back to smoking pretty regularly, you probably need to set a new Quit Date, review Steps 1 and 2 and start again at Step 3. The next chapter has more on learning from your relapse and reorganizing your efforts. Don't be discouraged. Remember what we've repeated often. The average successful quitter relapsed several times before getting it right. Relapsing doesn't mean you are a failure. Relapsing and learning from your mistakes and trying again are all part of successful quitting.

Progress Calendar

The calendar on page 160 is designed to chart your monthly progress. Be sure to make a photocopy and hang it up someplace where you're likely to see it several times each day.

At the bottom of the calendar, there's a contract for you to sign, in which you promise to become a permanent nonsmoker. As the months go by and you get used to being a nonsmoker, you may tend to forget about your campaign and the need to remain vigilant. Having a monthly checkpoint can help.

You'll see an empty circle at the bottom of each month. That's to help you count your savings! Remember, one of the rewards of not smoking is that you'll save money. Whether you smoked one pack a day or three, the savings add up. So at the end of each month, calculate how much money you've saved and write it on the calendar.

COUNT YOUR SAVINGS

If cigarettes are selling for about $2.00 a pack in your area, here's how much you'll save:

Period of Time	Packs of Cigarettes (not Smoked) Each Day				
	1	1-1/2	2	2-1/2	3
Day	$2.00	$3.00	$4.00	$5.00	$6.00
Week	$14.00	$21.00	$28.00	$35.00	$42.00
Month	$60.00	$90.00	$120.00	$150.00	$180.00
Year	$730.00	$1,095.00	$1,460.00	$1,825.00	$2,190.00

More Rewards

Each month on the calendar also has a space for a reward. You may want to reward yourself each week—you deserve it!—but even if you don't, be sure you plan a reward for yourself at least once a month. As we said back in Step 4, these rewards won't make you stay off cigarettes, but they give you a nice reminder every week or month—a reminder that you are doing something worthwhile for yourself and that you do need to stay vigilant.

Don't put off your reward because you feel it's too much trouble or it's making too much out of too little. Staying on your reward schedule can be a key reminder to stay with the rest of your plan.

So, do be sure to reward yourself. The kind of reward that will work best is up to you. But as the weeks go by, chances are that a variety of three kinds will be most effective: mental rewards, treats, and gifts.

Mental rewards involve giving yourself time to think about what you've gained by giving up smoking. For example, you can think about the fact that you're free of a habit that cost you a lot of time and money. A second example: feeling good about being a good role model for your children. A third example: thinking about the health benefits that come from not smoking.

Treats also cost little or no money. Examples are spending some extra time on a hobby, getting together with a friend you haven't seen in a while, or sleeping late on a weekend day.

Gifts do cost money, but they don't have to be expensive to be effective rewards. The only requirement is that they are things you enjoy. Gifts can include a new CD, a book about a special interest or hobby of yours, a fishing lure, a pair of running shoes, a plant—whatever appeals to you.

MENTAL REWARD DIARY

It's easy to lose track of our successes and the things we feel good about. Even with all the attention you've given to quitting, you will be surprised how easy it is to forget to give yourself a little credit. Try setting aside a little time each day—maybe before going to sleep or when you first get up in the morning or first get home from work— and write down some notes about why you feel good about quitting. Just writing down your thoughts will cause you to realize that you have more reasons for feeling good than you thought you had. So the little bit of time can really have a payoff.

After a while, you'll probably cut this down to every couple of days rather than every day, but do try to continue to write down your notes at least once a week. It's a satisfying way to keep some attention on your plan.

You can use some of the money you saved to reward yourself. Early in the month, write in the reward or rewards that you've planned for yourself.

MY SMOKE-FREE LIFE CALENDAR

Chart your progress for one year. Write the amount of money you've saved in the circle next to each month you stay off cigarettes. Write the reward you will give to yourself on the line provided for each month. Then, sign you're your name at the bottom.

January

Saved:
Planned Reward:

_____

February

Saved:
Planned Reward:

_____

March

Saved:
Planned Reward:

_____

April

Saved:
Planned Reward:

_____

May

Saved:
Planned Reward:

_____

June

Saved:
Planned Reward:

_____

July

Saved:
Planned Reward:

_____

August

Saved:
Planned Reward:

_____

September

Saved:
Planned Reward:

_____

October

Saved:
Planned Reward:

_____

November

Saved:
Planned Reward:

_____

December

Saved:
Planned Reward:

_____

I resolve to continue my **7 Steps to a Smoke Free Life** program for the entire year.

Signature_____   Date_____

COPY—CUT

Vigilant about Temptations

In order to stay on your course of becoming a nonsmoker, you'll have to keep vigilant and guard against the temptations that could cause you to slip up.

If only temptations would go away, now that you've stopped smoking! Unfortunately, they don't. Not for a while. In the first few months, when you see or taste a cup of coffee or make a telephone call, you may be just as likely to get an urge for a cigarette as you did when you were a smoker.

By the time you've been off cigarettes over two weeks, the frequency of your urges is going way down. But some urges can still be real killers. Here's one consolation: The worst is over! The nicotine is gone from your system, most physical withdrawal symptoms are sharply reduced, and the frequency of those urges and cravings is going down.

That means the cravings you're experiencing are coming from your mind, not from your body. Try not to be discouraged or frustrated by this. Habits you've had for years are not something that will disappear overnight. The important thing is to recognize where the urges are coming from and to use that knowledge to fight the craving.

THOUGHTS ARE NOT URGES

As the months go by, you'll start to notice that even your mental cravings are becoming more like thoughts than strong drives.

Ex-smokers who have been off cigarettes for a long time say they still have thoughts about cigarettes, but not pressing urges. It's a bit like what happens when you hear old hit songs. The music evokes thoughts of your high school days, and the friends you knew then—but you don't feel any urge to actually go back to cramming for exams and agonizing over acne.

Of course, some ex-smokers who want to boost their own egos often brag that they're still fighting urges to smoke every day. But they're usually just trying to make themselves appear strong, while frightening others from even attempting to quit.

Reevaluate Your Temptations

So how can you deal with these temptations, now that smoking is out of the question? Creative Alternatives and Do Power, of course.

Now is a good time to reevaluate your temptations and your plans for coping with them. As your physical cravings have decreased, you've probably noticed that the temptations that used to affect you may no longer be the ones that bother you now.

Cigarettes and cigarette packages are still likely to be your strongest temptations. You got rid of all your cigarettes when you quit smoking. But now's the time to do a double check of all the places where you used to keep them. The obvious places, such as cigarette boxes. And the not so obvious places, such as the side pocket of a suitcase. It's important to make sure you really got rid of every last one, because one of the easiest ways to fall off the wagon—especially when you are feeling confident that you have mastered your desire for cigarettes—is to come across a couple of leftover cigarettes.

Q U I C K   Q U I T   T I P :

Do a double check of all the nooks and crannies where you might have tucked cigarettes: seldom-worn jackets or handbags, glove compartments, etc. You don't want to be tempted in a moment of weakness.

Next, read through the list of common smoking temptations listed in the box below. Pick out the ones that you think are now most troublesome to you and write them in the blanks on the worksheet. Of course, add your own biggest temptations if they are not on the list.

For each temptation you list, write in a Creative Alternative, either from the list or one you've developed yourself.

Then, identify a Do Power strategy for each temptation.

When you're through, you'll have a pretty good, up-to-date plan for some of the temptations that still lie in wait for you.

TEMPTATIONS AND CREATIVE ALTERNATIVES

Temptation

▶Having an alcoholic drink
▶Watching TV
▶Getting ready for a meeting
▶Talking on the telephone

▶Drinking coffee
▶Finishing a meal
▶Taking a work break
▶The end of the workday

Creative Alternatives

▶Stretch and touch your toes
▶Do Deep Breathing Exercises
▶Do a crossword puzzle
▶Knit, crichet, embroider
    sew
▶Build a model plane,
    boat, train

▶Go for a walk
▶Exercise
▶Take a shower
▶Suck on a stirring stick
▶Chew sugarless gum
▶Doodle

Strategies

Example:

Morning coffee

Temptation

Creative Alternative:

*Do the cross word puzzle
from the paper rather than
smoking.*
Do Power: *Skip coffee at
home and have it at the
office where I can't smoke.*

Now, on the next page, you try it!

TEMPTATION #1   Creative Alternative:——————

———————————

——————————— Do Power:———————————

TEMPTATION #2   Creative Alternative:——————

———————————

——————————— Do Power:———————————

TEMPTATION #3   Creative Alternative:——————

———————————

——————————— Do Power:———————————

Avoiding Smoking Places And People

A strong Do Power strategy is to avoid smoking places as much as possible during your transition to becoming a nonsmoker. This includes:

▶ Smoking sections
▶ Bars, restaurants, canteens
▶ Bowling alleys and golf courses

It's not only places that present a problem, though, it's people—people who smoke, that is. Most relapses begin with a cigarette offered by another smoker.

You are vulnerable to the temptation to join in when someone else lights up. This is especially true when ex-smokers are feeling confident they have their smoking under control. A friend offers them a cigarette, they figure they can have just one, and so it goes. That's why it will really help during the next few weeks if you avoid people who smoke, even if they're your best friends. Also try to pass on social situations that involve smoking. It's bad enough when you watch one person light up, but watching five, ten, or more people smoke—well, you get the picture.

You might even make a list of your friends and acquaintances who smoke. Put your closest smoking friends at the top of the list, and your casual smoking friends and acquaintances at the bottom of the list. Then draw a line at that place on the list where your close smoking friends end and your casual smoking friends and acquaintances begin.

Of course, the object isn't to destroy your friendships. Rather, your goal should be to spend a little less time with your smoking friends, and a lot less time with casual friends and acquaintances who smoke.

A little Do Power can help here. Anticipating that you'll miss being with your friends who smoke, you might plan to talk to them on the phone, or meet them in a nonsmoking setting, say, at a movie, or even going for a walk together.

The Party

A lot of relapses occur in social situations. Drinking, talking with friends, feeling relaxed and maybe a little too confident about your smoking, or perhaps feeling a little shy and anxious, and being offered a cigarette—these can trip up the best of us.

DO POWER IN SOCIAL SITUATIONS

Of course, you can't avoid all social situations where people may be smoking. But you can get through them without smoking. Here are some Do Power strategies to keep those temptations from getting control.

1. Shortly before you get to the party, review in your mind your firm decision that you will not smoke, nomatter what.

2. Take some time shortly before the party to visualize yourself not smoking in key situations that are likely to occur. Think of what the place will look like. If it includes a meal, try to imagine what will be served. Practice saying, *out loud,* "No, thanks, I quit." This will help to internalize your resolve.

3. To make sure you don't feel anxious or like a wall flower, plan some things you'll talk about, perhaps a funny story you heard or an article you read in the newspaper.

4. Drink something nonalcoholic during the party or limit yourself to one drink.

5. Talk ahead of time to friends who will be there. Tell them you are concerned but determined, and ask them to give you encouragement during the party.

6. Ahead of time, use Positive Self-Talk to affirm your decision not to smoke.

Rehearsing As If It's Important

Whether you visualize your plan or just think it through, the more detailed you are, the more likely you will be to *do* what you want. Here's an example of a detailed plan:

"I see myself coming into the room and I'm not smoking. I'll say hello to John, Susan, and Kathy without smoking. I'll ask them about the parents' committee at the school. If Susan offers me a cigarette, I'll just tell her I quit. I know she'll understand—she probably won't light up around me. I'll tell her I appreciate this

*and that I hope that in another month her smoking won't bother
me anymore, or maybe she'll want to quit too. Once I get something to drink, I'll find Joe and Carol and talk with them
about the latest movie they've seen—they're always up-to-date
on that. . . "*

It requires some thought to work out all those details, but
that's just the point. The more thought you give it ahead of time,
the more likely you'll be able to stick with it when you actually
face the temptation.

But what if someone who knows you've quit smoking tries to
offer you a cigarette anyway, with a comment like "Aw, c'mon.
What are you trying to prove? Are you some kind of health nut?"

Think back to the Assertive Responses you learned about
in Chapter 3. You might say something like "No. I don't want
to be annoying about it to my friends. But I thought it over and
realize that not smoking is what I want."

ULTIMATE DO POWER PRIORITIES

But what if, despite all your precautions and all your assertiveness, you still
have trouble with your urges to smoke? What if they get stronger and
stronger, and you don't think you can hang on much longer? Just leave! Go
home. Or go for a walk until your smoking urges have quieted down.

Now, when I say that, you probably think, "Oh, that's silly. I can't leave
a party because I feel like a cigarette." Why not? You'd feel okay leaving
the party early if your baby-sitter couldn't stay late, or if you had to get up
very early the next morning to meet an important deadline.

Quitting smoking is important, too—clearly important enough to leave
a party for during the first weeks or months of becoming a nonsmoker.

More Creative Alternatives and Do Power for Cravings

▶ **Waiting it out.** When your craving is a mild one, it's often
possible to wait it out. After 5 or 6 minutes, the urge often fades
and disappears.

▶ **Reviewing your most important reasons for quitting
smoking.** Remember your Top 5 Reasons for Quitting Smoking. Now
is a good time to review them. Since you've been a nonsmoker for
awhile, some new reasons may have made their way onto your Top 5.

▶ **Talking yourself out of an urge.** You read about Positive Self-Talk in Step 6. Use this approach to get past an urge. Try telling yourself the following:

- "I'm doing really well. This urge won't throw me if I don't let it."
- "This isn't going to last. This will go away."
- "I really want a cigarette right now, but I'm not going to have one. Instead, I'm going to take a walk."

▶ **Thinking away the urge.** Recall some of the diseases related to smoking that meant the most to you. Then think how you have lowered your odds of getting them. Then say to yourself, "I will not smoke."

▶ **Relaxercise** and deep breathing. Keep at them!

QUICK QUIT TIP:

It is possible to talk yourself out of an urge to smoke. When you're hit with an urge, tell yourself: "Hey, this isn't going to last. This will go away." And it will!

A Quiz on Creative Alternatives and Do Power

Picture yourself in this situation: You've been behind your desk or behind the wheel of your car for hours. You're feeling cooped up and restless—the kind of feeling that had you reaching for one cigarette after another. Now that you're a nonsmoker, what will you do to deal effectively with these feelings? Think for a moment. Then say your answer silently to yourself.

If you said something like, "Stop and take a long stretch," or "Take a soda break," you're on the right track.

Here's another situation: Your car is in for service and you're waiting around until it's finished. It's taking much longer than you expected and you're getting really impatient. Before you quit, you used to keep yourself occupied by smoking. And indeed, there may be several people in the waiting area who are smoking. So what will you do? Again think for a moment, and then say the answer silently to yourself.

Did you think of something else to do, like running some errands? Or did you picture yourself taking a paperback book or magazine from your pocket and getting involved in reading? Maybe you had a deck of cards in your pocket and you decided to play solitaire.

You get the idea. Be sure to remember this approach during your daily activities. Whenever a situation or an emotion you're feeling creates an urge to smoke:

▶   Take a moment to think of something to do about it.
▶   Say what you're going to do, silently to yourself.
▶   Do it!

Meditation

Now that you no longer have cigarettes to take the edge off of stress, you may want to try meditation. Although meditation is associated with several spiritual traditions, this version is a simple, non-religious one. Here, meditation is simply training you to focus your attention in a way that releases tension. It feels somewhat like dozing, because it causes a drop in your breathing rate and your blood pressure.

Here's how to do it:

1.   Sit quietly in a comfortable position in a chair. Or you can sit cross-legged on a bed or on the floor if you like, but it's not necessary.
2.   Close your eyes.
3.   Consciously try to relax all your muscles as much as you can.
4.   Breathe through your nose, and each time you breathe out, say the word "one" (or choose another simple word).

Focus your mind on the word "one" as you're saying it. If ideas come into your head that distract you, just notice them a little and then bring your mind slowly and easily back to the word "one." Don't try too hard to focus your attention in any one direction. You want to go with what comes to mind, while you gently work your way back to "one."

Do the meditation exercise once or twice a day for 15 to 20 minutes in a place where you can be alone. Using meditation and the other breathing techniques will help you cope not only with tension related to quitting smoking, but with tension in general. In fact, you may find these techniques helpful even when your smoking days are long gone.

QUICK QUIT TIP

Drinking and Smoking *DO* Mix

About that drink you're carrying—best to make it non-alcoholic. A stiff belt is just what you *don't* need to cope with an urge to smoke. If you're feeling no pain, or even if you're just a little bit high, your judgment and your resolve can falter fast.

Stick with club soda on the rocks or ginger ale—two soft drinks that look like hard drinks.

If you feel you must have an alcoholic drink, try to limit it to one and maybe make it last by adding soda or some other mixer.

THOUGHTFUL MEDITATION

As you let thoughts come into your consciousness, you may find yourself mulling over current concerns, but in a more relaxed and open manner than when you "worry" about them.

Sometimes, you may experience new or fresh views of your concerns, seeing them in a broader light than when you're struggling with them. In meditation, you see the forest, not the trees.

As you meditate, you may find yourself having some new thoughts about why you quit smoking or why you feel good about it. The process encourages seeing connections among all the parts of your life and things going on around you—it's natural to see some new connections between quitting smoking and the rest of your world.

Don't Con Yourself into Smoking

A part of you is still wanting to get back on cigarettes. It may try all kinds of tricks to get you to take up smoking again. Perhaps you'll recognize your personal con artist in these typical situations:

▶ **Situation:** You're given a rush job just a few minutes after you get to work. It's got to be done by 4:30 or else. A voice inside you says, "This one's special. You can have just a few cigarettes today and then go back to nonsmoking tomorrow. Besides, I'll do better work if I smoke."

▶ **Situation:** You're at a meeting, and you're about to make a speech. You're nervous, and the voice inside you says, "This speech is important, and you don't get to do this very often. If having one or two cigarettes will help, they're justified."

Have you been hearing that little voice, too? At these times, it's important to remember that quitting smoking is hard and important. For example, one assertive response you could say to yourself in the first situation might be:

"This is a tough spot to be in. But I'm not going to waste all the time and trouble I took giving up smoking just because of one rush job. Besides, six months from now I won't remember this assignment, but I will be very happy if I'm still not smoking. When the urge for a smoke hits, I'll get up and stretch. If that doesn't work, I'll try sugarless gum."

In the second situation, you might think to yourself:

I know I can make this speech without a cigarette. Even though it's special, it's not as special as my getting off cigarettes. Not smoking is making me feel better physically and mentally. And who knows, I may impress those who realize I used to smoke."

Controlling Your Weight

That inner voice saying "I have to go back to smoking" may sound especially loud when you get on the bathroom scale in the morning. Have you been gaining weight? Many ex-smokers do. Indeed, concern about weight gain is a real hurdle for most people. It's the reason many smokers are afraid to quit. And when smokers do quit, if they gain weight, they often go back to smoking to lose weight.

But that *doesn't* have to happen to you! Smoking changes how your body stores fat. When you quit, your body starts to go back to normal for your age, sex, and height. That accounts for the pounds you may gain. It's simply an effect of the decreased level of nicotine in your body. You can't control this change in your metabolism. So try not to worry about your weight gain right away. Your first priority is to concentrate on staying off cigarettes. Don't forget that a few extra pounds are not nearly as bad for you as smoking.

After the first couple of weeks, you can start focusing on exercising more and eating better. We review some specific tips in the box in the next section, Eating Better.

Some scientists believe that getting off nicotine causes craving for sweet foods. If you're eating more high-calorie, sweet foods, nicotine withdrawal may be part of the reason. Food also tastes better now that you're not smoking. Eating gives you something to do with your hands. And for many people, eating is also an escape from boredom and tension. All of these work together to encourage you to eat more.

STAYING OFF THE WEIGHT AND SMOKING MERRY-GO-ROUND

You may quit smoking, gain five pounds, go back to smoking, lose the five pounds, quit smoking, regain the five pounds...

Here's how to get off the merry-go-round:

- ▶ Quit smoking for good.
- ▶ Work to recognize that the weight gain is less important than staying off the cigarettes. Consider buying some health books or magazines that will provide and reinforce healthy choices.
- ▶ Don't worry about eating less, concentrate on eating more healthily and exercising more.
- ▶ When you can cut back on calories without finding yourself tempted to smoke, you can start planning how to lose the weight.

In short, you need to solve the smoking problem first, and then work on the weight when you can do so without triggering strong urges to smoke.

QUICK QUIT TIP:

After you've successfully gone without smoking for a month or more, are you still gaining weight? It could be that you're reaching for food whenever you get the urge to smoke. Instead of eating, try drinking—that is, non-alcoholic beverages. Keep a glass of water, club soda, juice, or diet soda nearby throughout the day.

Eating Better

Before you turned the page, you may have been worrying "I know what's coming next—I'm going to have to go on a strict diet. Just what I don't need while I'm still battling the urge to smoke!" You're right. Restricting your calories is not what you need now.

So, the good news is: no diet. Instead, eat more of the healthy foods. Unless you've gotten into some really bad habits—like eating lots of ice cream every day—you don't have to worry about eating less of anything. Of course, by simply concentrating on eating better, you will fill up on good food and hopefully have less desire for fats and sweets.

Here's what to do:

▶ Eat more lean meat and fish. Lean meats such as veal, chicken, and turkey are low in fat and calories and high in vitamins and minerals. The same is true for fish.

▶ Eat more fruits and vegetables. The FDA advises that you "Strive for Five"—have at least five servings of fruits and vegetables each day.

▶ Eat less sugar. If you take in more sugar than the body needs, the excess sugar is converted into body fat. Sugar is an obvious ingredient in cookies, cakes, and candy. But it also hides in many canned and frozen convenience foods. Check the nutrition labels on the products you buy for glucose, sucrose and other sugars.

▶ Cut down on fat. Use low-fat milk, yogurt, and cottage cheese instead of whole-milk products. Trim fat from food. Broil, bake, or steam instead of frying foods in fat.

▶ Go easy on the booze. Alcohol doesn't provide nutrients, but it does provide a high dose of calories.

▶ Eat three square meals a day. Skipping breakfast and lunch won't help you control your weight, but it's liable to give you headaches, jitters, and a ravenous appetite that may lead you to binge or look for a cigarette. Eating three moderate meals through the day will make you feel better, will get your metabolism going better, and will probably result in your having fewer total calories than if you skip a meal or two.

▶ Eat the right snacks. Good choices are foods that take a long time to chew, like apples, unbuttered popcorn, carrots, and celery sticks.

▶ Cook with herbs and spices. That way, you'll use less butter, margarine, and fattening sauces.

▶ Start your meals right. Have a clear soup, or an "undressed" green salad, or a low-calorie drink (water, seltzer, tomato juice, tea) before eating a meal. It will help fill you up.

What you do—and don't do—is just as important as what you eat or don't eat. For example, *do* get lots of exercise. That will burn calories, cut stress, and make you feel good. Also, *do* eat when you're hungry, not when you're bored. And finally, when you're through eating, get up. *Don't* sit there thinking about dessert—or a cigarette.

Q U I C K   Q U I T   T I P :
When you're through eating a meal, get up. If you just sit there, you'll wind up thinking about dessert—or a cigarette.

Feeling Good about Yourself

You may be looking at your scale every day, and worrying about your weight. But have you been looking in the mirror? If not, take a look right now! Have you noticed any changes? Many ex-smokers notice that their color is better, their teeth are whiter, and their eyes are brighter.

And remember, what's happening inside you is even more important than what you see on the outside. Your body has already started to repair the damage that smoking has caused.

So you should be feeling pretty good about yourself! After all, quitting smoking is no small potatoes. For lots of folks, it's as important an event as starting a new job, or buying a house. What's more, quitting smoking can give you a greater sense of being in control of your life.

Discontinuing Nicotine Replacement

As your sense of control increases, you may want to think about discontinuing the use of any nicotine replacement products you've been using. As time goes on since your last cigarette, you'll no longer need to rely on nicotine gum, patches, sprays or inhalers.

When you start thinking about getting off sprays or medication it may be a good time to check in with your doctor. He or she will be glad to hear about your progress and might be able to help you plan getting off the nicotine replacement.

If you have been using nicotine gum or nicotine patches—both of which are sold without a prescription—you can begin the weaning process by yourself. Most people follow this approach:

Nicotine Gum: Use nicotine gum every day for at least two to three months after quitting. If you have successfully stayed off smoking for that time, you will be able to gradually reduce the number of pieces of the gum you use each day. When you get down to just one or two pieces a day, you can stop using it. But continue to carry some with you for a few more weeks, in case of an emergency situation which might tempt you to smoke.

On the following page are some techniques to use when you are ready to wean yourself off the nicotine gum medication.

Design your plan so that you will be completely free and confident of your freedom from nicotine in six months. For most smokers, that means starting to cut down on nicotine gum after three months of use.

Nicotine Patches: Many people prefer the simplicity of a single strength patch. But, some patches come in different sizes and shapes. The larger the patch, the more nicotine it delivers through the skin. Many smokers start with the strongest patch. Then after several weeks, they can switch to a medium strength patch for a few weeks, and possibly a lower strength patch for the last few weeks.

Patches are available for either six-week or ten-week treatment periods. They are usually not meant to be used for more than three months. Although some people are able to stop using nicotine patches at this point without a tapering-off period, a gradual dose reduction is often recommended. If you are using a brand of patches that come in several dosage levels, taper off by switching to the next lower dose for two weeks. If an even lower dose is available, switch to that for your last two weeks. If you are using a single-strength patch, you can try wearing the patch for only half a day, or skipping every other day, then skipping two days, and so on.

Whichever tapering approach you decide on, be sure to err on the side of using the replacement for a longer rather than a shorter period of time. Generally, the entire course of nicotine patch use and gradual tapering-off should take no more than fourteen to twenty weeks.

Is it hard to give up the nicotine patch after so much time? Studies have shown that it is much easier to give up the patch than it is to give up cigarettes, for two reasons:

▶ One of the reasons smoking is so attractive is that the nicotine reaches the brain in about seven seconds. With the patch, the nicotine level in your body stays relatively constant day after day. There is no immediate "hit," so little craving develops.

▶ In smoking, all the things that you are doing while you smoke become linked to the nicotine "hit." Talking on the phone, drinking coffee—they all develop strong links to the nicotine. Since you put on the patch only once a day, and receive a steady stream of nicotine, no links are developed.

QUICK QUIT TIP:

Tips for Weaning from Nicotine Gum

1. Reduce one piece a day for five days. If you feel any withdrawal symptoms during the week, don't decrease the next day. Instead:

- ▶ Stay at that level for one week.
- ▶ Then, begin to decrease again.
- ▶ After five days of decreasing, stay at that level for one week.

2. Repeat the above procedure until you get to one or two pieces a day. Stay at one or two a day for one week, and then quit.

3. As you cut down, cut the pieces in half or replace one or more pieces with regular sugar-free gum.

4. Start chewing the pieces for only half the time. This will help you break the chewing habit, if you need to.

Nicotine Nasal Spray and Nicotine Inhaler: You may have been getting nicotine administered via a nasal spray or by the newest method, an inhaler. Both of these are prescription products. Your physician will give you instructions on weaning yourself from these. Recommended strategies include:

▶ Use only half a dose at a time
▶ Use the spray or inhaler less frequently
▶ Skip every other dose for several days. Continue to skip more doses on succeeding days

Prescription Medication: If you have been taking the "**non-nicotine pill**," Zyban, which is available only by prescription, your doctor may have provided only a seven or eight week supply. Some studies have found that extending treatment beyond eight weeks does not increase the pill's effectiveness. So, your doctor may want to wean you off the non-nicotine pill at this point, if you have successfully stopped smoking. However, longer treatment may be advised if your cravings are not yet controlled well enough to guard against a possible relapse.

Am I Done Yet?

By the time you've reached this point in the book, you've probably asked yourself more than a few times, "When can I relax about this whole business of stopping smoking?" The answer is "Not yet!"

There's still more to do, but you deserve tremendous praise for your successful progress so far. Think of how far you've come:

▶ In Step 1, you gained an understanding of your habit and your addiction to nicotine, and you learned to identify your smoking temptations.
▶ In Step 2, you gained the resolve to decide to quit.
▶ In Step 3, you developed your personalized quitting plan.
▶ In Step 4, you learned how to break up habits, deal with temptations, and get the cooperation you needed in preparation for your Quit Day.
▶ In Step 5, you took the big step—your Quit Day—and you successfully managed the first 24 hours.
▶ In Step 6, you worked on managing symptoms of physical and psychological recovery from nicotine during your first two weeks as a nonsmoker, and you learned how to treat slip-ups as an emergency.

▶ In Step 7, this final step, you learned long-term strategies for staying vigilant against smoking tempatations, and for keeping your weight under control

Congratulations! You've accomplished a lot.

Reaching Six Months

When you get to six months after your Quit Date, you obviously have a lot to be proud of. Even though we've talked earlier about people having trouble recognizing their own accomplishments, you probably won't have any trouble with this one, or with feeling great in another six months when you make one year. So enjoy it. You've accomplished something that was hard but very, very worthwhile.

Now is the time for making one more list. For this one, there is no form. You make it up. Put down what you think are the most important things you want to keep in your mind to make sure you don't get in trouble with smoking in the future. Maybe it's some of your Top 5 Reasons for Quitting. Maybe it's a key Creative Alternative or Do Power tactic. Maybe you've begun walking every day, have come to love it, and want to make sure you never give it up. Maybe you've learned new ways to cope with anxiety or sadness, or maybe you've learned some skills for being less shy or more assertive. Whatever, write yourself a note or make yourself a list of the key ideas you want to keep in mind to protect your great accomplishment.

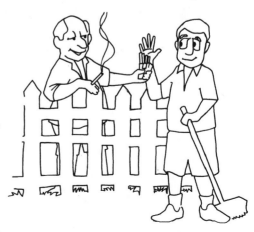

Practice going without cigarettes. Keep practicing to stay quit.

PART THREE

Perfecting the Nonsmoking Habit

CHAPTER 12

How to Cope with a Relapse:
What to do now

Quitting smoking takes practice. It takes more practice for some people than for others. In fact, almost everyone who tries to quit slips up once or twice and smokes a cigarette.

Having a couple of cigarettes is one thing. It's a slip-up. As discussed in Step 6, quitters need to be *determined* not to have even a single puff. But, on the other hand, they need to recognize that *slips are common* and not get too dejected if they have one.

Having a couple, then a couple more, then a couple each day—that's quite another thing. Before you know it, you're back to smoking at least a few cigarettes every day. It's a judgment call, but at that point you've probably gone from slip to relapse.

If you realize that you have relapsed, don't get down on yourself. It doesn't mean you've failed. Give yourself a break. Forgive

---

**RELAPSE IS NOT FAILURE—
IT'S PART OF YOUR CAMPAIGN TO QUIT
SUCCESSFULLY**
Remember: **The average successful quitter
relapses 2–4 times before succeeding.**

---

yourself! Millions of people who have quit smoking don't succeed on the first try, or even the second or third try. Many of these smokers still end up quitting for good. So each time you try to quit is a real step forward. A recent Harris survey of 1,002 smokers found that those who had tried to quit made an average of five unsuccessful attempts. Most of these smokers who tried to quit started smoking again within a month's time. Many said they began smoking again because they faced a stressful situation and needed a cigarette to cope. Being around others who smoke was also a common reason for resuming the smoking habit. Are either of these situations what happened to you?

How to Get Back on Track

If your most recent attempt didn't succeed, what can you do about your smoking now? You have two basic choices:

1. If you have smoked just a few cigarettes for two or three days, and you feel you had made some good progress toward successfully quitting, treat this setback as a temporary slip.

STOP SMOKING IMMEDIATELY!

THROW AWAY ALL YOUR CIGARETTES!

And right now, reread the section in Step 6 of this **7 Steps to a Smoke-Free Life** program under the heading "What happens if I slip up?" (page 148).

Remember, this is an **EMERGENCY!** Act **NOW!**

2. If you have gone back to smoking several cigarettes a day for more than a couple of days, you may conclude that you have relapsed. At this point, you need to decide whether to re-start your quitting program immediately, or take a few days' break to get your thoughts together.

Just as we talked about in Steps 3 and 4, what's important is that you quit with determination and clarity. You may do better if you take some time to gather your thoughts, review your reasons and plans for quitting and start over. If so, you can skip to the section, Starting Over on page 193. But if you think you want to try to lick this thing now, keep reading.

BEWARE THE INNER CULPRIT

Remember the Inner Culprit we discussed back in Step 6? This is the part of you that might like to conclude that, "Gee, my case is hopeless. You gotta' go somehow. I might as well just relax and enjoy life and stop punishing myself this way."

The Inner Culprit ignores the part of you that knows:

▶ Slips and relapses are often part of the path to success.

▶ Half of all smokers—millions of heavy smokers—have quit.

▶ Quitting is more important than the other things you do for your health.

▶ Most important: You really do *want to do it!*

Consider Sticking with It

You should do an immediate re-start, to get right back on track. You have invested considerable time and effort in your success thus far. You may not have finished your plan, but you have made a good start! Don't give up now! After all, your time off cigarettes has already cleared much of the nicotine out of your system. You've survived the worst days of nicotine withdrawal. And you've already had some good practice in Do Power to cope with smoking triggers and in using Creative Alternatives to give you substitutes for cigarettes when you get the urge to smoke.

Read through the next few pages and see if it doesn't help you make up your mind to quit again.

Fast Track to Re-Quitting

Every cigarette you don't smoke, every time you say "No!" is a small victory. Every small victory helps you beat your old smoking habit. Practice makes perfect. If you slipped up, it means you didn't quite handle a temptation you faced. It doesn't mean that you are a failure or that you are addicted and can't quit.

So before you go any further, add up your victories:

▶ On the next page, check off the days you went without cigarettes.

▶ Also record the days on which you smoked one, two, or more cigarettes.

▶ On the next line, indicate what went wrong, if you can. Examples might be "friend offered me a cigarette" or "stressful work situation."

▶ On the next line, indicate what steps you could have taken that might have helped you to avoid smoking in that situation.

The goal is to pinpoint what went wrong each time you slipped and had a cigarette. Forget guilt and blame. Instead, focus on what caused the slips and what you will do differently next time. For example, you may find that your slips occurred only in the evening, when you were home relaxing and watching television. A Creative Alternative might be to have some substitutes ready while watching television in the evening, perhaps busy work or some hobby you can do at the same time, or perhaps some reasonably healthy snacks.

A Do Power strategy might be to keep yourself busier at this time of day, at least until you're more practiced in your nonsmoking habit. You could plan social engagements for the evening hours, or work on a hobby instead of watching television.

Or try Visualization. Close your eyes and get the situation in your mind: It's evening. You're at home, and you're not smoking. What do you see yourself doing?

QUICK QUIT TIP

Practice to Perfect

If you intend to exercise four days a week but miss a few, if you intend to "cut out sweets" but enjoy some candy at holidays, if you vow to balance your checkbook every month, but sometimes don't get it done until the tenth of the following month, you're still doing pretty well.

What's hard about quitting smoking is you need to practice until you get it perfect.

Long-term, successful ex-smokers almost never puff. Virtually all of them feel that "it's easier to have none than one."

MY SMOKING CESSATION VICTORIES
AND SLIP-UPS

Put a check mark on the days when you were smoke-free. Put an "X" on the days when you smoked. Describe what went wrong, and what coping steps might have helped you avoid smoking in that situation.

	Sun.	Mon.	Tues.	Wed.	Thurs.	Fri.	Sat.	Total # Victories
Wk. 1:	____	____	____	____	____	____	____	_____

Slips: What went wrong? _____
What might have helped? _____

	Sun.	Mon.	Tues.	Wed.	Thurs.	Fri.	Sat.	Total # Victories
Wk. 2:	____	____	____	____	____	____	____	_____

Slips: What went wrong? _____
What might have helped? _____

	Sun.	Mon.	Tues.	Wed.	Thurs.	Fri.	Sat.	Total # Victories
Wk. 3:	____	____	____	____	____	____	____	_____

Slips: What went wrong? _____
What might have helped? _____

	Sun.	Mon.	Tues.	Wed.	Thurs.	Fri.	Sat.	Total # Victories
Wk. 4:	____	____	____	____	____	____	____	_____

Slips: What went wrong? _____
What might have helped? _____

Specific Plans

Now make a list below, including the temptations from the previous page and other difficult triggers you're likely to face tomorrow. Then write out a plan for how you'll manage them tomorrow. Don't worry about the next day, or the next week. Right now, you're going to take it one day at a time. So concentrate on tomorrow:

COPING WITH TOMORROW'S TEMPTATIONS

List the temptations you are likely to face tomorrow or over the next few days. Describe your plan for dealing with each.

Temptation	**My planned action**
_____	_____
_____	_____
_____	_____
_____	_____
_____	_____

When tomorrow arrives, look at this list so you'll know in advance how you can handle each temptation. Try to use as many of the tactics in this book as possible—Creative Alternatives,

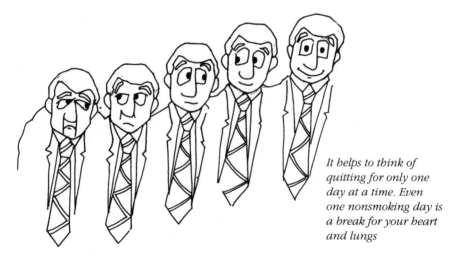

It helps to think of quitting for only one day at a time. Even one nonsmoking day is a break for your heart and lungs

Do Power, Relaxercise, Visualization—until you find one that really works for you. If you slip up and smoke a cigarette, don't give up. You'll do better when the next temptation occurs, if you just keep practicing.

If you're having trouble thinking of new things to do when cravings hit, check the list of alternatives below.

WHAT TO DO WHEN THE CRAVING COMES...

Eat something!
▶ A low-calorie snack: fruit, veggies.

Distract yourself!
▶ Whistle. Sing. Brush your teeth. Take a shower. Call a friend.

Analyze!
▶ Do you think you need a cigarette as a reward to relieve boredom, or after an extended period of concentration? Find another way to take a break.

Move!
▶ Get up and walk around. Take a drink of water. Do relaxation exercises. Stretch, yawn, do deep knee bends, touch your toes, shrug your shoulders.

Think!
▶ Think of quitting as an act of love—for those you care about. It's also a gift to yourself.

Mental Preparation

When you first decided to quit smoking, you began the process of *learning* to be a nonsmoker. You thought about the benefits smoking had offered you—such as stress relief, weight control, social acceptance. You also tallied the negatives—the health risks, the expense, the loss of control over your life. Then you identified alternative activities you could use to replace smoking in your life. The next step was to begin practicing those alternatives.

A FUNNY THING ABOUT MOTIVATION

We think of motivation as something that happens to us. "Joe is really motivated."

But motivation isn't something that happens. It's really something you do. You can practice being motivated!

What this really means is that if you keep your reasons for wanting to quit in your mind, think about them a few times a day, challenge your Inner Culprit, use Positive Self-Talk, and practice Visualizing yourself being successful, you'll find that all your reasons for wanting to quit get stronger in your mind. Then they'll be more help to you in quitting for good.

You've had *some* practice over the past few weeks, but you're still learning. This learning stage will continue until you get really "good at" nonsmoking. That usually takes at least several weeks, but often two or three months. So if you've stumbled recently, it doesn't mean you can't accomplish your goal. It simply means you'll have to continue in the intensive learning stage for at least another month or two.

When a sports team stumbles and loses a few crucial games, the coach usually calls for increased practice sessions. But as coaches also know, there's another element needed for a winning performance: *mental preparation.* You probably remember practicing Positive Self-Talk in Step 6 (see page 140). That's the kind of mental preparation you need more of.

Continue to monitor your "inner voice." You'll probably will go back to smoking if you tell yourself too often that you're deprived. Talk to yourself! Talk about the benefits of not smoking. (Take out your Top 5 Reasons for Not Smoking card and reread it now.) Remind yourself that you are healthier now that you are a nonsmoker. Remember, this has been a great accomplishment. You will begin to like yourself as a nonsmoker. It's in your power to let either deprivation or determination take over.

What Positive Self-Talk can you use? Start with "I can do it! I can keep myself from smoking!"

When you're in a difficult situation and feel like smoking, tell yourself, "The urge will pass whether I smoke or not."

If you're at a social gathering and someone tempts you by offering you a cigarette, think to yourself, "I can say 'No!' I feel good when I stand up for what I believe in."

QUICK QUIT TIP

What to say to myself when I want to smoke:

1. "The urge will pass whether I smoke or not."
2. "I'm not going through the pain of quitting again!"
3. "I like my body when I'm not smoking."
4. "I'll distract myself until the urge passes."
5. "I deserve credit for quitting smoking."

If you've ever participated in sports, you understand the value of this mental preparation. Just as athletes get mentally ready for a big event, you'll have to "psych yourself up" for the smoking challenges you'll face each day.

Visualization is another tool athletes use. They "see" themselves scoring the winning run or making the winning basket. In the same way, you can visualize yourself as having achieved the goal you have in mind: becoming a nonsmoker. Then act as if it were true.

Here's how to do it:

1. Choose a positive phrase you are willing to repeat to yourself each day.
2. Visualize yourself in a new situation and continue to repeat that phrase until you smile and begin to believe it.

Can you think of a phrase you might use? Perhaps one of these examples will work for you:

▶ "I feel better since I've stopped smoking."
▶ "I feel a lot more in control of myself."
▶ "I am so glad that my world no longer revolves around cigarettes."
▶ "There's nothing that could ever get me to go back to smoking."
▶ "I'm doing this because I finally decided I want to."

Are Your Family and Friends Encouraging You?

Just as athletes rely on their team members and encourage each other, don't forget that you have a team, too. Now that the going's gotten rough, it's time to call on your team—the family and friends who will cooperate and encourage you in your "big game." Take time to talk with your family and friends.

At this point, you probably have a better idea of who is really helpful in guiding you around temptations, or just understanding what you're going through. Follow these leads. Maybe you'll arrange a meeting for lunch or phone calls or just a calm walk together after dinner. Whatever style works for you, think about getting more of their company— and encouragement!

> "I called a friend when I had trouble avoiding a cigarette. I asked her to talk me out of it or keep me company to distract me. It worked!"
> —Veronica, age 40

If you have one key family member or friend whom you've looked to for help, review how that's gone. Because you've slipped up in your nonsmoking plan, you may have hesitated to keep in touch with him. Were you afraid of discouraging him? Or maybe you've been too embarrassed to call and admit your problems. If he cares about you, he'll understand and want to be helpful. But chances are good that your key person will be a lot more understanding than you may fear.

Make that call! If your friends or family members are exsmokers, they will know how good it feels and will be happy to give you all the encouragement they can. And if they had trouble quitting, too, they can make you feel understood. Maybe you can put your heads together and come up with a few new strategies that could help you.

Family Obstacles?

Finally, think about your family situation. Under the best circumstances, your family members will be rooting for you all the way. But perhaps your spouse or your parents are smokers. They may resent your efforts, or feel guilty about not trying to quit with you.

If this has been a problem in your family, it could be the reason you've had trouble staying quit. Studies show, for example, that those who fail to quit or who relapse are more likely to be married to a smoking spouse and/or to have many friends and family members who smoke.

Try to think of your quitting as separate from their smoking. It's their right to smoke and it's your right to quit. You can't make your spouse or family members quit smoking. So focus on cooperation and support from other family and friends who don't smoke.

But of course you don't want to avoid the people you love. Try to separate talk about your quitting from talk about their smoking, and make the talk cooperative, not angry:

"I know I will drive you nuts if I preach to you about why you ought to quit. And you'll drive me nuts if you tell me that my quitting isn't fair to you. So, for a while, we probably need to leave each other alone about smoking and concentrate on other things together."

You can still expect your family to cooperate with your quitting. Remember Healthy Selfishness. You might negotiate with them about:

- ▶ Limiting their smoking in specific situations that are heavy temptations for you, like in the kitchen after dinner. You can't ask them not to smoke, but you can identify situations in which it would be a big help if they didn't.
- ▶ When it's possible, ask them to smoke outside the house, perhaps on the front porch, back patio, or terrace. But it's their house, too, so you may want to take a walk when they're smoking. Try to keep this friendly and cooperative, not demanding.
- ▶ When they do smoke inside, ask them to smoke in rooms that have windows or fans to send the smoke outside.
- ▶ Work together to come up with a plan about guests smoking in the house.
- ▶ Ask them not to smoke in the car.
- ▶ Ask them to sit with you in nonsmoking areas.

Asking Too Much?

Some of this may seem like a lot. Of course, when you think about it, quitting smoking is such an advantage for your health, it doesn't make too much sense for others to do anything that will stand in your way. But, attitudes and family patterns change slowly. Also, your smoking relatives may be so conscious of their own wishes to stop smoking—whether or not they acknowledge it—that asking them to limit their smoking, or even the fact that you're quitting, may annoy them. So you will need to cooperate and compromise with your family. One approach that may be helpful is to stress that you are just asking them to cooperate with you for the first month or so, while you get used to life without cigarettes. It's not that you are asking them never to smoke in front of you again.

What Else Can I Do for Myself?

Smokers who are thinking of quitting often worry that they'll be too stressed out, or that they'll gain too much weight. Did this happen to you when you weren't smoking? If so, go back and reread the sections on stress management (see page 142) and weight control.

Exercise is an effective remedy for both problems. So if you haven't been getting regular exercise, think about perhaps thirty minutes, three times a week for a session of moderate exercise. Even going for a daily walk for fifteen or thirty minutes may be great exercise for you. It's a stress fighter, and a Creative Alternative in a time when you might otherwise light up.

You don't need elaborate equipment to exercise. You don't need to join a gym (although that could be a nice idea, if it appeals to you.) Just get out and walk, or ride a bicycle, or go for a swim. The idea is to have fun—*active* fun.

One other tool you can use to help yourself is to plan rewards and celebrations. Right now, you may tend to be a bit hard on yourself. Maybe you had thought about rewards for your progress, but if you've had some slips, you may really think there's not much to celebrate now.

This is just the time to consider a different approach. Maybe you need to lighten up and go easy on yourself. You probably have made a lot more progress than you would have bet a month or two ago. Maybe you need to treat yourself to half of something or part of something you like, to symbolize that you've made progress, even if you haven't accomplished all you set out to. If you make it through the rest of today or tomorrow smoke free, that's reason enough for at least a small reward. See if you can get into a more generous spirit with yourself and give yourself all the credit you deserve for the progress you've made.

Forget about words like failure or will power. You haven't failed, you're still practicing. Use rewards to help you set small goals. Don't let small victories go by unnoticed. It reminds you that you've done far too much work to go back to smoking.

Starting Over

If you feel you need a break before tackling quitting again, that's not a problem. Remember, the average person who succeeds as a nonsmoker may quit a few times and then relapse before finally getting it right. You can learn from your relapse, regroup, and get it right!

Although you're not ready to quit right now, don't put the thought out of your mind. Before you forget, take a few notes about your experience this time, so you'll have something to build on next time. Here are some questions to ask yourself:

- ▶ What was the best part of your effort?
- ▶ What did you do that was most helpful?
- ▶ As you were working on quitting, what reasons for quitting and benefits seemed most important or meaningful to you?
- ▶ What was the biggest problem you faced in trying not to smoke?
- ▶ What problems turned up that you didn't expect?
- ▶ Were you bothered by a major life change or stress that is unlikely to recur in the future?
- ▶ Where did you get cigarettes when you slipped up? Did someone give you one? Or did you find a hidden stash at home or at the office?
- ▶ When did you move from a simple slip to smoking two or more cigarettes a day? What happened?
- ▶ You know yourself best: What do you think is most important for you to remember the next time you quit?

Here are some other factors to consider in trying to learn from your effort to date:

Timing. Perhaps the time of year wasn't right for you. If you quit in the summer this time, when you take vacations and have lots of free time, you might want to plan your next Quit Date for the winter, when your time and activities are more structured.

Quitting Group. Some people enjoy and do well working together with others who are also trying to quit. Next time, you might try joining a group program. Your local chapter of the American Lung Association can give you the schedule for the *Freedom From Smoking®* clinics in your area.

Nicotine replacement. If you did not use a nicotine replacement product this time—nicotine gum, patches, nasal spray or nicotine inhaler—you might consider doing so next time. Some of these products are available over-the-counter, without a prescription.

If you did try nicotine replacement and it didn't help enough, ask yourself whether:

▶ You should have used it longer, or used a stronger dosage.
▶ You used it correctly—check the directions for using nicotine replacement in Step 3.
▶ You may have relied too heavily on the nicotine replacement and not enough on doing things toorganize your quitting, maximize your motivation, and combat temptation. Remember, nicotine replacement is not a "magic bullet." You may want to consult your doctor or pharmacist on this. You might also ask them if other medications might be helpful for you, like the non-nicotine pill we described in Step 3.

Doctor's advice. Just because you don't need a prescription for nicotine gum or nicotine patches, doesn't mean you shouldn't consider seeing your doctor. If you didn't check with the doctor this time, you might plan to do so the next time you're ready to quit. You may be advised to use one of the prescription nicotine replacement products, such as the nicotine spray or inhaler. If a low mood or stress were troubling factors for you, that's something to discuss with your doctor, too.

Weight gain. Did increased weight cause you to go back to smoking? That's a common occurrence. You might speak with a nutritionist to plan a weight-control diet. Or join a spa or gym and work on a program of regular exercise. That way, you'll have weight control tools ready the next time you quit.

Exercise. We've stressed exercise a lot. It can be a real help. If you haven't exercised much, it may have been hard to get it started at the same time you were trying to quit. You might want to start an exercise plan now, before quitting again. Then, when you quit, you will have exercise to fall back on.

QUICK QUIT TIP

Special Hint on Exercise

If you start exercising before you quit, even just walking four or five times a week, you will find your enjoyment of exercise increases after you quit. This is the automatic benefit that quitting will have on your wind and vitality. So getting into exercise ahead of time is a good way to build an automatic reward into the first couple of weeks after you quit.

Moods and Relapses. Many people relapse when they are feeling anxious or sad. If that's what happened to you, you might go back to the sections on stress management (see page 142) or check out the next chapter on coping with moods.

Lots of people control their moods by smoking. When they quit, they can be surprised that they are having feelings of real sadness or anxiety that they hadn't realized before. It shows how effective nicotine is in blocking our feelings. If this has happened to you, you might want to speak to your doctor about using the medication described in Step 3, which helps with depression in the same way nicotine does. Or, on your own or with your doctor's advice, you might decide to see a counselor (a psychologist, psychiatrist, or social worker) who can help you work on what may be troubling you That way quitting will be easier for you next time.

Finally, take the time to think about the pros and cons of

quitting smoking. When you try again, you want to be clear on your own reasons for wanting to quit. And, you want to be clear that you want to quit, not that someone or something is driving you to it. A half-hearted, renewed attempt to quit is likely to end in relapse, which runs the risk of lowering your motivation and confidence. Give your quitting the attention it and you deserve. Start fresh—go back through Steps 1 and 2, so that you will be clear that you want to, and confident that you will, quit smoking. You've already made a lot of progress and learned a lot. You **can** do it!

CHAPTER 13

Keeping Frustration from Frustrating Your Plans to Quit

As you may have discovered, smoking was often automatic in your life—so automatic that you were unaware of the moods, thoughts and feelings that prompted you to smoke. Step 6 discussed some of the feelings, especially sadness and anxiety, that may have been triggers for lighting up, and may still be temptations for relapse.

But you can also feel like smoking when you are frustrated: at work, with family or friends, with your spouse or with your children. This chapter will give you some ideas for dealing with these frustrations. It discusses skills that can improve your interactions with friends, help you cope with problems in families and relationships, and become more assertive and effective in expressing your feelings

Advantages of Getting to Know Your Feelings

Continuing to refrain from smoking will be easier if you keep in touch with your feelings, likes and dislikes, worries, and irritations. Start taking your feelings into account. Before you might have said, "I feel like having a cigarette." Now you have learned to ask yourself which feeling is leading you to that. Learning to be more in touch with what you are feeling should be one of the greatest benefits of quitting smoking. It can help you improve other areas of your life as well.

Social Skills

Feeling lonely or uncomfortable with others may have been one of the reasons you used to smoke. Each of us has had the experience of not knowing how to approach someone, what to say first, or how to get a conversation going again when it stalls. The following tips can help make your social interactions smoother:

1. Make sure you're *involved* in conversation. Don't just think about what impression you're making. Focus on the others. Show you're interested in their views. Ask questions. Listen to the answers. Find things to agree with the others about, or to compliment them on.
2. Watch others who seem particularly good at the skills you've decided to work on. You're bound to pick up some pointers. Tell them about times you feel frustrated or inadequate and see what they suggest. We all have these feelings sometime. Other people are likely to be pleased to tell you how they handled the problem.
3. Ask friends to observe how you're doing on the skill you choose to develop and to give you feedback on your progress.
4. Think of situations in which you wish you had acted differently, and also some in which things went well for you. Use these as models to help you decide what to do in future situations.

Talking with others takes skill. If your conversations don't go well you're likely to end up with anxious, angry, or sad feelings—internal cues for cigarettes. Go over the following Questions to Ask Yourself to make conversations go better. Little changes in how you approach conversing can, over time, make you a lot more comfortable. Then, the feelings that make you smoke will become less of a problem.

QUESTIONS TO ASK YOURSELF: MAKING CONVERSATION GO BETTER

TALKING

▶ Do you talk too softly or in a monotone?
Are your personal or critical comments too loud?

▶ Would talking more slowly make you easier to understand?

▶ Do you talk too slowly, so your listeners tend to finish your sentences?

▶ Is your choice of language colorful enough without being overly familiar or vulgar?

BODY LANGUAGE

▶ Do you stand too close or too far from those you're talking with?

▶ Is your body too stiff? Or are you often waving your arms and overusing facial gestures?

▶ Do you avoid eye contact, or make people feel you're staring at them?

SENSITIVITY

▶ Are you being sensitive to the needs of others?
Do you turn people off by turning discussions away from their concerns and to your own interests or problems?

▶ Do you make others feel like just part of your audience? Do you let others speak?

▶ Do you frequently interrupt?

Family and Relationship Skills

When your personal life is running smoothly and you have the cooperation and support of those close to you, it's easier to make changes in your own behavior. But when you're having trouble communicating with your spouse or guiding your children, changing your own habits can seem overwhelming. Improving some aspect of your family life may really help you remain a nonsmoker.

Family members can make emotional demands that challenge your efforts to stay off cigarettes. Not knowing how to make family interactions meet your own needs and those of the rest of the family can be a real problem. The example below may seem familiar:

> *After dinner Sherry announced she was going for the regular after-dinner walk she'd started since she quit. Matt had been patient for three weeks, but he was tired of being stuck with the dishes every night. He blew up at Sherry and they argued.*

Couples like Sherry and Matt might avoid confrontation if they communicated their feelings and needs to each other more clearly. Recognizing that Matt was tired of cleaning up, it might have been helpful if Sherry told Matt how much his doing the dishes had helped her to stay off cigarettes, and how much she appreciated it. She could have suggested a schedule for going back to sharing this chore. She might also have suggested doing the dishes together, and then going for a walk together.

Here are some hints on communication skills that have helped others.

1. Ask yourself what you really want. Is it really what just happened that is bothering you? Do you really want to confront your partner or other family members about it? Or are you feeling hurt or unappreciated in some other, more subtle way? Communicating that "I need some special help this week" can be more pleasing and is more likely to be successful than an attack or accusation that others are not doing their fair share.

2. Close the gap between what you mean and what they think you mean. When the people you're talking with respond inappropriately, assume they've misunderstood, not that they don't care. Clarify what you mean. Make sure there isn't a misunderstanding.

3. When trying to resolve a particular issue, avoid getting off the subject and bringing in other complaints. This happens when

partners let their needs and wishes and frustrations get tangled in a knot. Instead of solving one question, they keep drifting into others, which makes them tired and frustrated. Stick to the topic at hand and discuss it honestly.

4. Avoid "mind reading." Often we assume that we understand all the thoughts, feelings, and needs of those we know well. Frequently this is wrong and leads the other person to feel you're not tuning in. Check your assumptions by listening carefully and asking questions.

5. Don't counter each point the other person makes with your own parallel complaint. If your partner complains that you failed to take the garbage out, don't answer by complaining about your partner's forgetting to feed the cat. If everything others say leads you to say, "yes, but..." people will not feel as though you've understood them.

6. In discussions of problems and emotions in a relationship, it helps to start each sentence with an "I." This forces you to focus on what you feel and tends to keep you from attacking your partner. If you express your frustration honestly ("I felt hurt when you read the paper during breakfast and didn't talk to me.") it's less likely that your partner will try to make you feel badly.

Better communication skills can help improve aspects of your home life and make it easier to be a non-smoker. By learning to express your feelings, to ease tensions before they mount up, and to resolve disagreements without unpleasant arguing, you can avoid feelings that might otherwise send you in search of cigarettes.

Communicating with Children

Avoiding conflict with your children while you're trying to quit smoking is as important as avoiding conflict with your spouse. At some period in their lives, many children use "NO" as the main word in their vocabulary. Children who routinely refuse instructions this way may have learned that disobeying gets them their parents' attention.

They've also learned that refusal works. Parents often stop asking children to do things if each request leads to argument or has to be repeated. But you can change this pattern; if you focus on praising children when they're being cooperative, and cut off interactions when a child is disobedient.

Here are some suggestions:

1. Give your children attention when they are cooperative. Let them know you notice when they are being helpful. If refusal habits are strong, have a plan to reward cooperation systemati cally. Points or gold stars earned for daily cooperation could be redeemed for a favorite TV show, a special dessert, or a long bedtime story. You must implement such a system consistently to make it work.

2. Communicate clearly. Make sure your children know what you expect of them and exactly how they should cooperate. Let them know what the benefits of cooperation will be. Just like your spouse, they can't read your mind—although sometimes it seems they can.

3. Draw your children into making plans with you. Let them know how you're feeling and what you need. If you tell them hon-estly that you are especially tired or that you may be a little on edge because you've recently quit smoking, they may be more eager to help. Also give them some choices, so they feel they have some control. If you want them to pick up their rooms, for example, you can say, "What would you like to do first? Put your clothes in the hamper or put your blocks in the toy box?" Also you might propose a fun activity to look forward to doing together after the housework.

4. Don't give your attention to refusals. Once you've made a clear and reasonable request, don't keep repeating it. If the child doesn't cooperate, you may decide to punish him mildly. For instance, you might postpone a planned activity until you get cooperation. To break the connection between your child's refusal and your paying added attention, you might send her to another part of the house, away from you and things she enjoys. But this should be done calmly, not in anger. You are only trying to break up this pattern, not make the child suffer. After five or ten minutes you could bring the child back and repeat your original request. These more controlled ways of dealing with refusal should help you keep your own emotions under control, lessening the urge to smoke in frustration.

Even if refusal isn't a big problem with your children, the suggestions above can help you gain their cooperation with your efforts to quit smoking. Let them suggest ways to help. Don't hesitate to ask your family for help. Your need to quit smoking is important and they should cooperate.

The skills of being a good partner and a good parent have much in common. Remember the main points: to be clear in your own mind about what you want, and to make your wants known to others. Be calm and consistent and avoid getting side-tracked into less relevant issues.

Asserting Yourself and Your Feelings

Most of us feel that sometimes we can't say what's on our mind or that we can't reach out to people. There are many reasons for this—we're shy, anxious to be polite, worried about others' reactions, trying to avoid an argument, or afraid of rejection.

You may be thinking "I don't have trouble saying what's on my mind." But now that you have quit smoking you may find that the feelings of frustration or annoyance you used to handle with a cigarette now make you feel like a time bomb. So even if you haven't had a problem with this in the past, you may find you do now. Consider this example:

> John fumed as he stormed out for his morning break. His supervisor had just asked him to stay after work to put in some extra hours on a project. The boss requested this all too often, and this time meant John was going to have to miss watching his oldest son pitch in a ball game for the third time in a row. "Why am I always the one who has to stay?" John thought as he contemplated lighting a cigarette. "After all, Denise is responsible for getting this project done, too. Why doesn't he ever ask her to work late?"

What can John do instead of turning to cigarettes?

Communicate Feelings. John can tell the boss how much his son was counting on him to show up for the ball game. He shouldn't assume that people know the extent to which certain requests are difficult for him.

Suggest Alternatives. John can suggest that Denise stay this time, pointing out that she shares responsibility for getting this project completed.

Of course, pointing out alternatives won't always get you out of the office on time for the ball game. In general, though, speaking up (calmly) will make you feel less frustrated and powerless.

We think of assertiveness too much as only standing up for ourselves. But people who have trouble letting others know they are bothered by something may also have trouble letting people know they like something. Again, try thinking of assertiveness more in terms of communicating your feelings—positive or negative—rather than as sticking up for yourself.

PRACTICAL STEPS IN BEING ASSERTIVE

Try thinking of these steps before and after asserting yourself:

1. **Identify your feelings.**
2. **Figure out what others are feeling.**
3. **Express your understanding of the other person's point of view.**
4. **Express your feelings.**
5. **Ask for the other person's thoughts.**
6. **Suggest a possible solution or compromise.**
7. **Ask for the other person's response or suggestion.**

Here's an example:

Thoughts to yourself: I really want to do the best job I can, but my boss and my co-workers are feeling rushed and anxious about meeting the deadline. I need to reassure them that I'm aware of the deadline. Okay, I think I'm ready to explain this.
You say: "You know, I really do want to make sure we make the deadline, but I also want to make this job the best it can be. I wonder if there is any way I can revise it a bit without throwing us off schedule. What do you think?"
They answer: "Well, we've got to get something to the client today, but I can arrange for you to look it over one more time at a later date."

You think: Great, they heard me. They're trying to be cooperative.

You say: "Okay. I can help get it done now, and you'll make sure I have a chance to look it over again later. That should be okay, right?"

They answer: "Yes, great. Thanks for understanding that we need to make this deadline."

WHAT ASSERTIVENESS IS

Assertiveness is: expressing yourself comfortably without hurting others or denying their needs

Assertiveness covers: a range of positive as well as negative feelings—from being able to ask someone (politely) not to smoke, to saying "I love you."

Assertiveness is also a lot about details. What works in one situation won't work in another. Are there particular times when you have trouble saying how you feel? For example, saying how you feel and what you want early in an interaction can prevent an unpleasant ending to the conversation. Here are more suggestions for paying attention to these kinds of details:

DETAILS TO REMEMBER

To be more assertive, remember that you want to express your own feelings and invite cooperation. You're not looking for a fight. Focus on three aspects of what you say and do.

1. *What you say:* Are you describing your feelings or attacking the other person? You want to get your own feelings out where others can recognize and react to them. Attacking the other person will only draw attention away from your feelings and to the fact that you seem angry. Ask yourself if you've listened to the other person and show that in what you say.

2. *How you say it:* Consider how you make or don't make eye contact, your posture and gestures, the timing of what you say. Tone of voice, facial expression, and even how closely you stand to the other person all make you come off as confident and cooperative, or as passive and unsure of yourself, or as aggressive and challenging.

3. *The situation you are in:*
- What is your relationship to the other person?
- How direct you can be is probably different for a member of your own family than for a total stranger.
- Where are you?
- What may work in private may not work when you are part of a larger group or out in public with strangers.
- What led up to this point?
- Whether you come off as calm and confident depends a great deal on what has already been said. If you already made your feelings known and were ignored, you may need to be strong in your next statement. On the other hand, if the other person probably doesn't even know what's bothering you, being too strong may "blast them out of the water."

What's the Difference Between Being Assertive and Being Aggressive?

Don't confuse being assertive with being aggressive. Of course, we don't want to be pushy and obnoxious, always insisting on having things our way. You should see your needs and desires as important, but you also need to recognize the needs and desires of those you're relating to. Assertiveness seeks balance between your needs and theirs. If you always feel out of balance, you need to become more assertive, not more aggressive.

Further Thoughts and Further Sources

Developing friendships, cooperating in families, and putting yourself forward in a way that enhances your relationships rather than antagonizing others are all very complicated. Occasionally, people write about how to do better in these areas as if it is simple. It surely is not.

So, these thoughts just scratch the surface. There are many other points of view and approaches that can also be helpful. Should you want to pursue some of these issues in further detail, books in the following areas might be helpful:

- ▶ assertiveness
- ▶ social skills
- ▶ improving relationships between spouses
- ▶ child management

Additionally, many people at some point in their lives seek counseling to help them come out of their shells, learn how to deal more effectively with their family members, or become more assertive and do a better job of representing their own interests. As we noted in Step 6, if you think you would like to talk to a professional about any of these issues, you can find a psychologist, social worker, or psychiatrist through your local mental health association, your doctor, or possibly your friends.

CHAPTER 14

A New Breath of Life

You've made some significant changes in your life by using this book. This final chapter looks at how you may have changed, the goals you want to keep in mind for the future, and how you can apply the skills and confidence you have gained to many other areas of your life.

New Ways of Looking at Yourself

Quitting smoking is a funny thing. In a sense, it is very simple—you simply stop putting those little white cylinders to your lips. But it is also very complicated. You had used smoking to cope with all sorts of challenges, from feeling energetic in the morning, to getting out of a bad mood during the middle of the day, to calming down before trying to go to sleep. Smoking was woven into many different areas of your life.

Having quit, you have learned to look at yourself, your habits, and your emotions in a whole new way. And because quitting smoking was so hard, you may feel a particular sense of pride or satisfaction in your ability to have done it. You deserve this pride!

One of the reasons this is especially true is because quitting smoking requires the vigilance we talked about in Step 7. In contrast, think about exercise. If you exercise four times a week for a few weeks, then miss a couple of days, then get back into it, and then miss a week; but, over the course of a year, average two, three, or four days of exercise per week, you will be doing pretty well. This is not true with smoking. You have found that you needed to stay off cigarettes *every* day in order to stay quit. This has required an extraordinary commitment on your part.

Frequently, meeting one challenge makes us feel more confident in our ability to meet others. This certainly applies to quitting smoking. What you've accomplished is a lot harder than most of the goals people set for themselves, such as to exercise more, eat healthier food—or get their taxes done early. Now that you feel like a success with smoking, you may want to take on some other challenges that you've been hesitant about.

NEW CHALLENGES WAITING FOR YOU

Most of us have a mental list of things we would like to do, or change, in our life. Just in case you need some suggestions, here are a few to stimulate your creative juices. As with so much in this book, you need to figure out for yourself what's right for you:

HEALTH:

▶ Regular examinations appropriate to sex and age

▶ Pap tests and mammograms for women

▶ Prostate exam for men

▶ Cholesterol or blood pressure screening, depending on your age and family history

▶ Improve your diet, your exercise habits, your sleep (seven hours a night minimum), your drinking patterns, or your stress management

FAMILY:

▶ Spend more time with your spouse and children

▶ Encourage better health habits in your family—Could your family learn that celebrating a birthday by taking a family hike beats going to a fast food restaurant?

PERSONAL:

▶ Take up that old hobby you let go, whether it's playing a musical instrument, crafts, or stamp collecting

▶ Join a club or take an evening course through the local high school or college

▶ Get out those drafts of short stories you started ten years ago and finish one—submit it to a magazine.

If you do take on some new challenges, many of the strategies you've used to quit smoking may be helpful. Of course, there is no equivalent of the nicotine patch for staying up-to-date with household bills, but a lot of what we've talked about does extend to other situations.

Begin by looking at the motivation behind the choices you are making. *Why* do you want to learn Italian, run a 10K race, institute "date night" with a spouse? Very few people are motivated by things they feel they "should" or "ought" to do. Make sure your choices are things you are doing for yourself—or that you have solid external reasons for your decisions. Being clear about your motivation will help carry you through.

Start off with Do Power. Most of the problems that stand in the way of your goals can be looked at from the perspective of the three key components of Do Power:

▶ Specify the problem you are trying to solve, the goal you are trying to achieve.
▶ Creative Problem Solving. Be clever in figuring out how you can solve your problem or reach your goal. Make sure your plan is right for you.
▶ Do it—implement the plan you develop.

For example, you might plan to pay the monthly bills after the kids are in bed, but then, you find that you're always too tired and just want to relax by that time of the evening. It may be sufficient to decide that you will write one check every evening before dinner. If you did that, all the bills would stay nicely paid. Taking it one step further, it might be helpful to sort the mail and keep your checkbook and records in one location to facilitate writing one check each evening before dinner.

Another one of your goals may be to improve your social life. Some innovative and fun options might be:

1. Join a club or team, but only if the activity is one you actually like or want to learn.
2. Invest some time in a hobby or volunteer job. Make sure it is one that will really give you satisfaction, not just fill your time.
3. Invite some friends, or new people you'd like to get to know, over for dinner.

Your Physical Health

Now might be a good time to look at some physical changes you'd like to accomplish. Building that commitment to healthier living into your daily experience can help you feel more committed to other ways in which you can live more healthfully.

Diet and Exercise

If you gained more weight than you wanted to in quitting, now may be the time to begin focusing your attention on losing it. Caution: it's still more important to stay off cigarettes than to lose the ten or even twenty pounds you may have gained. So if working on losing weight causes you more urges to smoke, drop off that merry-go-round until you can diet without looking for a cigarette.

Step 7 included a lot of good information on exercise and eating more healthily. This is probably worth reviewing at this time.

Diet is an especially good area in which to apply many of the same tactics for quitting smoking presented in this book. Remember how, before you quit, you systematically stopped smoking in the situations that caused the strongest urges? You can do the same thing with some of the situations that currently cause food cravings. For example, if you make it a rule never to eat while watching TV, while talking on the telephone, while driving in the car, or in whatever other situations currently make you "hungry," you will find that these situations pretty quickly lose the power to drive your cravings.

The Do Power strategies we talked about can help with a lot of eating that is out of control. Identify and specify your most troublesome temptations, figure out clever ways to change those situations so they will be less tempting, and implement your plan to see how it works. For example, if nibbling on leftovers is a problem for you, try planning meal preparation to eliminate the leftovers. If the cookies your children like drive you nuts, negotiate to keep other types of cookies in the house and ask your children to get their favorites at school. *Remember that these are only suggestions. What works well for one person may be a dud for another. You'll have to be creative to come up with your own Do Power strategies.*

Your weight loss efforts will also benefit from some rewards. Set goals for yourself and plan rewards that will make working toward them a bit more enjoyable. Here are two key hints:

1. Set your goals in terms of changes in eating habits. For example, decide to eat at least five servings of fruits or vegetables at least five days in the week, rather than deciding to lose a certain number of pounds. You don't need to be in a rush to lose weight. As dietitians have said for years, focusing on changing eating habits rather than losing weight is the best bet in the long run.
2. Don't make your reward a food treat. One of your goals is to learn to enjoy and relax with things other than food.

Going to the Doctor

Make sure you tell your doctor you have quit smoking. Don't be bothered if the doctor hasn't remembered you were trying. Most doctors' records aren't organized with a convenient place for noting smoking status, so keeping track of your quitting may be hard for your doctor. That's why you should bring up the subject. There are several good reasons for this. First, the fact that you've quit may help your doctor and you discover how being a nonsmoker can improve other problems for which you are treated. Your doctor might also want to change or adjust some of your medications now that you're no longer smoking.

Second, if you've gained some weight, you want to make sure the doctor knows it's "for a good cause." Especially if you have diabetes, hypertension, or a history of heart disease, it's important for the doctor to know your weight gain has come about from quitting smoking. Otherwise you may be pressured to lose it too soon, which could jeopardize your new status as a nonsmoker.

Another reason to tell the doctor is to encourage the two of you to take other steps to improve your health. Doctors love working with patients who *do things* to help themselves. When your doctor finds out you've quit smoking, he or she will be eager to work with you further to improve your health.

But of course, the best reason to discuss all this is so that your doctor will shower you with praise! Be prepared to be embarrassed. Really, most smokers say that they'd like to quit for their health. You probably had that as one of your reasons, too. Well, being able to tell your doctor that you feel confident you'll be a nonsmoker for the rest of your life is a moment you've been waiting for. Enjoy it.

Encouraging Others to Quit

If you are trying to tell someone you care about how much you would like them to quit, you might try a simple statement like: "I really like (or love, or care about) you and want to have a lot of time with you. But I'm afraid smoking could take you away much too soon." They won't be insulted by your telling them you'd like to spend more time with them. And the statement of your fear of losing them makes your point without making them feel you are telling them what to do. You might end with a simple offer of help, "I'd be willing to do whatever I can to help if you want to try it." But make sure it doesn't sound like you are nagging.

If they look the other way when you announce proudly that you've made it three months without a cigarette, you'll need a subtle approach. Try telling them four things:

1. You would never try to push them to quit.
2. You really were unsure about it, but now you are glad you quit.
3. What got you serious about quitting was realizing that smoking is so much more dangerous than all the other things we do to ourselves.
4. You'd be happy to talk to them about it, if they ever thought that would be helpful.

So be kind to smokers. Most—about 90%—would like to quit and wish they'd never started. Our goal (see, you're one of us, now) is to help them quit. Some are ready to receive a book like this. Some need a lot more coaxing before they're even ready to think about it. Try to remember this as you deal with smokers you know. If they are interested in giving it a try, give them this book.

Clearing the Air for Everyone

You may have become so energized by your experience with quitting smoking that you want to direct some of that energy toward preventing today's young people from starting to smoke in the first place. If so, the American Lung Association welcomes your help in our grassroots tobacco-control initiatives. ALA volunteers around the country are working to keep cigarettes out of the hands of children. Call your local American Lung Association at 1-800-LUNG-USA (or find the office nearest you in the resources section at the back of this book) or visit our Web site (http://www.lungusa.org) for the latest news on the American Lung Association's tobacco-control initiatives.

Last Words

I'd like to take this opportunity to say on the page what your body is surely telling you as well: Congratulations.

You have tackled something incredibly difficult. Your self-esteem and confidence should be soaring. I hope you are feeling proud, and very happy.

You have taken the time to learn numerous skills—Do Power, relaxation, and most important, recognizing what you really want and working to achieve it. All of these can be helpful in many other areas of your life. In addition, you have learned personal and interpersonal communication skills that can improve the quality of your life. These skills will help you bring renewed energy to important things you can do with your life, your children, your world. That's the most important reward for quitting smoking. Enjoy it.

Quit Smoking Resources

NATIONAL OFFICE
American Lung Association
1740 Broadway
New York, NY 10019-4374
(212) 315-8700
http://www.lungusa.org
America Online Keyword: ALA
The American Lung Association offers
a wealth of how-to-quit information
online, from the latest news to chat
groups and message boards.

GOVERNMENT RELATIONS Office
American Lung Association/American
Thoracic Society Washington Office
1726 M Street NW, Suite 902
Washington, DC 20036-4502
(202) 785-3355
By dialing 1-800-LUNG-USA from any-
where in the country, you are routed
automatically to your local American
Lung Association.

ALABAMA
ALA of Alabama
900 S. 18th Street
Birmingham, AL 35205
(205) 933-8821

ALASKA
ALA of Alaska
1057 W. Fireweed Lane, Suite 201
Anchorage, AK 99503-1736
(907) 276-5864

ARIZONA
ALA of Arizona
102 W. McDowell Road
Phoenix, AZ 85003-1299
(602) 258-7505

ARKANSAS
ALA of Arkansas
211 Natural Resources Drive
Little Rock, AR 72205-1539
(501) 224-5864

CALIFORNIA
ALA of California
424 Pendleton Way
Oakland, CA 94621-2189
(510) 638-5864

ALA of Alameda County
295 27th Street
Oakland, CA 94612-3894
(510) 893-5474

ALA of Central California
4948 N. Arthur
Fresno, CA 93705
(209) 222-4800

ALA of the Central Coast
174 Carmelito Ave.
Monterey, CA 93940
(408) 373-7306

ALA of Contra Costa-Solano
105 Astrid Drive
Pleasant Hill, CA 94523-4399
(510) 935-0472

ALA of the Inland Counties
441 Mac Kay Drive
San Bernardino, CA 92408-3230
(909) 884-5864

ALA of Los Angeles County
5858 Wilshire Blvd., Suite 300
Los Angeles, CA 90036
(213) 935-5864

ALA of Orange County
1570 E. 17th Street
Santa Ana, CA 92705
(714) 835-5864

ALA of the Redwood Empire
1301 Farmers Lane, Suite 303
Santa Rosa, CA 95405
(707) 527-5864

ALA of Sacramento-Emigrant Trails
909 12th Street
Sacramento, CA 95814-2997
(916) 444-5864

ALA of San Diego & Imperial Counties
2750 Fourth Avenue
San Diego, CA 92103
(619) 297-3901

ALA of San Francisco & San Mateo
Counties
2171 Junipero Serra Blvd., Suite 720
Daly City, CA 94014-1980
(415) 994-5864

ALA of Santa Barbara County
1510 San Andres Street
Santa Barbara, CA 93101-4104
(805) 963-1426

ALA of Santa Clara-San Benito
Counties
1469 Park Avenue
San Jose, CA 95126-2530
(408) 998-5864

ALA of Ventura County
2073 N. Oxnard Blvd., Suite 400
Oxnard, CA 93030-2964
(805) 988-6023

COLORADO
ALA of Colorado
1600 Race Street
Denver, CO 80206-1198
(303) 388-4327

CONNECTICUT
ALA of Connecticut
45 Ash Street
East Hartford, CT 06108-3272
(860) 289-5401

DELAWARE
ALA of Delaware
1021 Gilpin Avenue, Suite 202
Wilmington, DE 19806-3280
(302) 655-7258

DISTRICT OF COLUMBIA
ALA of the District of Columbia
475 H Street NW
Washington, DC 20001-2617
(202) 682-5864

FLORIDA
ALA of Florida, Inc.
5526 Arlington Road
Jacksonville, FL 32211-5216
(904) 743-2933

ALA of Central Florida, Inc.
1333 W. Colonial Drive
Orlando, FL 32804-7133
(407) 425-5864

ALA of Gulfcoast Florida, Inc.
6170 Central Avenue
St. Petersburg, FL 33707-1523
(813) 347-6133

ALA of South Florida, Inc.
2020 S. Andrews Avenue
Ft. Lauderdale, FL 33316-3430
(954) 524-4657

ALA of Southeast Florida, Inc.
2701 N. Australian Avenue
West Palm Beach, FL 33407-4526
(561) 659-7644

GEORGIA
ALA of Georgia
2452 Spring Road
Smyrna, GA 30080-3862
(770) 434-5864

HAWAII
ALA of Hawaii
245 N. Kukui Street, Suite 100
Honolulu, HI 96817
(808) 537-5966

IDAHO/NEVADA
ALA of Idaho/Nevada
6119 Ridgeview Court, Suite 100
Reno, NV 89509
(702) 829-5864

ILLINOIS
ALA of Metropolitan Chicago
(Chicago and Cook County)
1440 W. Washington Blvd.
Chicago, IL 60607-1878
(312) 243-2000

ALA of Illinois
#1 Christmas Seal Drive
Springfield, IL 62703
(217) 528-3441

ALA of Central Illinois
922 N. Sheridan Road
Peoria, IL 61606-1910
(309) 672-2290

ALA of DuPage & McHenry Counties
1749 S. Naperville Road, Suite 202
Wheaton, IL 60187
(630) 260-9600

ALA of North Central Illinois
402 Countryside Center
Yorkville, IL 60560

INDIANA
ALA of Indiana
9410 Priority Way West Drive
Indianapolis, IN 46240-1470
(317) 573-3900

IOWA
ALA of Iowa
1025 Ashworth Road, Suite 410
West Des Moines, IA 50265-6600
(515) 224-0800

KANSAS
ALA of Kansas
4300 Drury Lane
Topeka, KS 66604-2419
(913) 272-9290

KENTUCKY
ALA of Kentucky
4100 Churchman Avenue
Louisville, KY 40215
(502) 363-2652

LOUISIANA
ALA of Louisiana, Inc.
2325 Severn Avenue, Suite 8
Metairie, LA 70001-6918

MAINE
ALA of Maine
122 State Street
Augusta, ME 04330
(207) 622-6394

MARYLAND
ALA of Maryland
1840 York Road, Suites. K-M
Timonium, MD 21093-5156
(410) 560-2120

MASSACHUSETTS
ALA of Massachusetts
1505 Commonwealth Avenue
Brighton, MA 02135-3605
(617) 787-5864

ALA of Greater Norfolk County
25 Spring Street
Walpole, MA 02081-4302
(508) 668-6729

ALA of Middlesex County
5 Mountain Road
P.O. Box 265
Burlington, MA 01803
(617) 272-2866

ALA of Western Massachusetts
393 Maple Street
Springfield, MA 01105
(413) 737-3506

MICHIGAN
ALA of Michigan
18860 W. Ten Mile Road
Southfield, MI 48075-2689
(248) 559-5100

MINNESOTA
ALA of Minnesota
490 Concordia Avenue
St. Paul, MN 55103-2441
(612) 227-8014

ALA of Hennepin County
4220 Old Shakopee Road #101
Bloomington, MN 55437-2951
(612) 885-0338

MISSISSIPPI
ALA of Mississippi
353 N. Mart Plaza
Jackson, MS 39206-5316
(601) 362-5453

MISSOURI
ALA of Eastern Missouri
1118 Hampton Avenue
St. Louis, MO 63139-3196
(314) 645-5505

ALA of Western Missouri
2007 Broadway
Kansas City, MO 64108-2080
(816) 842-5242

MONTANA
[See ALA of the Northern Rockies]

NEBRASKA
ALA of Nebraska
7101 Newport Avenue, Suite 303
Omaha, NE 68152
(402) 572-3030

NEVADA
[See ALA of Idaho/Nevada]

NEW HAMPSHIRE
ALA of New Hampshire
456 Beech Street
Manchester, NH 03103
(603) 669-2411

NEW JERSEY
ALA of New Jersey
1600 Route 22 East
Union, NJ 07083-3407
(908) 687-9340

NEW MEXICO
ALA of New Mexico
216 Truman NE
Albuquerque, NM 87108
(505) 265-0732

NEW YORK STATE
ALA of New York State
8 Mountain View Avenue
Albany, NY 12205-2804
(518) 453-0172

ALA of Central New York
1620 Burnet Avenue
Syracuse, NY 13206
(315) 422-6142

ALA of Finger Lakes Region
1595 Elmwood Avenue
Rochester, NY 14620
(716) 442-4260

ALA of the Hudson Valley
35 Orchard Street
White Plains, NY 10603-3397
(914) 949-2150

ALA of Mid-New York
311 Turner Street, Suite 415
Utica, NY 13501-1731
(315) 735-9225

ALA of Nassau-Suffolk
225 Wireless Blvd.
Hauppauge, NY 11788-3914
(516) 231-5864

ALA of Western New York
210 John Glenn Drive, #3
Buffalo, NY 14228
(716) 691-5864

NEW YORK CITY
ALA of Brooklyn
165 Cadman Plaza East, Rm 300
Brooklyn, NY 11201-1484
(718) 624-8531

ALA of New York
(Manhattan/Bronx/Staten Island)
432 Park Avenue South, 8th Fl.
New York, NY 10016
(212) 889-3370 Manhattan
(718) 966-6700 for Bronx and Staten
Island

ALA of Queens
112-25 Queens Blvd.
Forest Hills, NY 11375
(718) 263-5656

NORTH CAROLINA
ALA of North Carolina
1323 Capital Blvd., Suite 102
Raleigh, NC 27603
(919) 832-8326
(800) 892-5650

NORTH DAKOTA
ALA of North Dakota
212 N. 2nd Street
Bismarck, ND 58501
(701) 223-5613

NORTHERN ROCKIES
ALA of the Northern Rockies
825 Helena Avenue
Helena, MT 59601
(406) 442-6556

OHIO
ALA of Ohio
1950 Arlingate Lane
Columbus, OH 43228-4102
(614) 279-1700

OKLAHOMA
ALA of Oklahoma
2805 E. Skelly Drive, Suite 806
Tulsa, OK 74105
(918) 747-3441

OREGON
ALA of Oregon
9320 SW Barbur Blvd., Suite 140
Portland, OR 97219-5481
(503) 246-1997

PENNSYLVANIA
ALA of Pennsylvania
6041 Linglestown Road
Harrisburg, PA 17112-1208
(717) 541-5864

ALA of Central Pennsylvania
6041 Linglestown Rd.
Harrisburg, PA 17112-1208
(717) 541-5864

ALA of Lancaster & Berks Counties
630 Janet Avenue
Lancaster, PA 17601-4584
(717) 397-5203

ALA of the Lehigh Valley
2121 Cityline Road
Bethlehem, PA 18017-2100
(610) 867-4100

ALA of Northeast Pennsylvania
738 South Maine Avenue
Scranton, PA 18504
(717) 346-1784 or 343-0987

ALA of Northwest Pennsylvania
352 W. 8th Street
Erie, PA 16502-1498
(814) 454-0109 or
(800) 352-0917 in local areas, outside
Erie County

ALA of Southeastern Pennsylvania
525 Plymouth Road, Suite 315
Plymouth Meeting, PA 19462
(610) 941-9595

ALA of South Central Pennsylvania
488 W. Market Street
York, PA 17404
(717) 845-5864

ALA of Western Pennsylvania
Cranberry Professional Park
201 Smith Drive
Cranberry Township, PA 16066
(412) 772-1750

PUERTO RICO
Asociación Puertorriqueña del Pulmón
P.O. Box 195247
San Juan, PR 00919-5247
(787) 765-5664

RHODE ISLAND
ALA of Rhode Island
10 Abbott Park Place
Providence, RI 02903-3700
(401) 421-6487

SOUTH CAROLINA
ALA of South Carolina
1817 Gadsden Street
Columbia, SC 29201-2392
(803) 779-5864

SOUTH DAKOTA
ALA of South Dakota
1212 W. Elkhorn Street, #1
Sioux Falls, SD 57104-0218
(605) 336-7222

TENNESSEE
ALA of Tennessee, Inc.
1808 West End Avenue, Suite 514
Nashville, TN 37203
(615) 329-1151

TEXAS
ALA of Texas
5926 Balcones Drive, Suite 100
Austin, TX 78731-4263
(512) 467-6753

UTAH
ALA of Utah
1930 South 1100 East
Salt Lake City, UT 84106-2317
(801) 484-4456

VERMONT
ALA of Vermont
30 Farrell Street
South Burlington, VT 05403-6196
(802) 863-6817

VIRGINIA
ALA of Virginia
311 South Blvd.
Richmond, VA 23220-5705
(804) 355-3295

ALA of Northern Virginia
9735 Main Street
Fairfax, VA 22031-3798
(703) 591-4131

VIRGIN ISLANDS
ALA of the Virgin Islands
P.O. Box 974
St. Thomas, VI 00804
(809) 774-8620

WASHINGTON
ALA of Washington
2625 Third Avenue
Seattle, WA 98121-1213
(206) 441-5100

WEST VIRGINIA
ALA of West Virginia
415 Dickinson Street
Charleston, WV 25301
(304) 342-6600

WISCONSIN
ALA of Wisconsin
150 S. Sunny Slope Road, Suite 105
Brookfield, WI 53005-6461
(414) 782-7833

WYOMING
[See ALA of the Northern Rockies]

Additional Resources
These organizations also provide
information on smoking and how to
quit.

Action on Smoking and Health
2013 H Street
Washington, DC 20077-2410
(202) 659-4310

American Academy of Otolaryngology
Head and Neck Surgery (AAOHNS)
One Prince Street
Alexandria, VA 22314
(703) 836-4444

American Cancer Society
1599 Clifton Road, NE
Atlanta, GA 30329
(404) 320-3333

American Heart Association
7272 Greenville Avenue
Dallas, TX 75231
(800) AHA-USA1 (242-8721)

Centers for Disease Control and
Prevention
National Center for Chronic Disease
Prevention and Health Promotion
Office on Smoking and Health
Mailstop K-50
4770 Buford Highway NE
Atlanta, GA 30341-3724
(800)-CDC-1311

National Cancer Institute
Bethesda, MD 20894
(800) 4-CANCER (422-6237)

National Heart, Lung, and Blood
Institute
Building 31, Room 4A21
Bethesda, MD 20892
(301) 496-4236

National Institute on Drug Abuse
Drug Abuse Information and
Treatment Referral Line
11426 Rockville Pike, Suite 410
Rockville, MD 20852
(800) 662-4357
(800) 662-9832 (Spanish)
(800) 228-0427 (hearing impaired)

For pregnant women:
American College of Obstetricians and
Gynecologists
409 12th Street, SW
Washington, DC 20024
(202) 638-5577

ACKNOWLEDGMENTS

Many Lung Association staff and volunteers have contributed to the development of ALA Freedom From Smoking® programs over the past twenty years. The late Roger Schmidt spearheaded the development of ALA's smoking activities. Stephen Ayres, M.D., and William Anderson, M.D. provided key volunteer support for the development of programs. Margaret Kane, Richard Straub, and Shane MacDermott developed the original Freedom From Smoking group program curriculum. Anne Davis, M.D. and Susan Rappaport, M.P.H. directed a volunteer and staff effort to develop and test the Freedom From Smoking self-help program. Since then, Sharon Jaycox-Daitz, M.S., Glen Morgan, Ph.D., Barbara Rimer, Ph.D., Tracy Orleans, Ph.D., Victor Strecher, Ph.D., Harry Cando, Ph.D. have assisted in further program development. Throughout this time, Karen Monaco, M.A. has provided invaluable staff leadership to development of ALA's programs.

A number of current and former colleagues and students of Edwin Fisher, Ph.D. have contributed to smoking research projects from which material in this book has been drawn. These include : Cynthia Arfken, Ph.D., Zev Ashenberg, Ph.D., Don Bishop, Ph.D., Wendy Auslander, Ph.D., Marti Bonte, Ph.D., Timothy Brown, M.A., Ross Brownson, Ph.D., Marion Capella, M.A., Rodney Coe, Ph.D., Mark Cook, Ph.D., Eric Crouse, Ph.D., Jerome Cohen, Ph.D., Jim Davis, Ph.D., Thomas DiLorenzo, Ph.D., Carolyn Dresler, M.D., Jane Grady, Ph.D., Leonard Green, Ph.D., Debra Haire-Joshu, Ph.D., Andrew Heath, Ph.D., Robert Hill, Ph.D., Jeanette Jackson-Thompson, Ph.D., Andre Jacobs, Ph.D., Randi Joffe, Ph.D., Steven Kurtz, Ph.D., Tami Levit-Gilmore, Ph.D., Michael Lowe, Ph.D., Karen Lucas, Pamela Madden, Ph.D., Joni Mayer, Ph.D., Amy Newman, Ph.D., Elana Newman, Ph.D., Denise Podeschi, Ph.D., Howard Rachlin, Ph.D., Gabrielle Reed, Ph.D., Heather Rehberg, Ph.D., John Rohrbaugh, Ph.D., Kathryn Rost, Ph.D., John Schulenberg, Ph.D., Vanessa Selby, Ph.D., Walton Sumner, M.D., Diane Weber, R.N., Teresa White, Ph.D., Kevin Whitney, J.D., and Sheryl Ziff, Ph.D. Special thanks to Glen Morgan, Ph.D. and Walton Sumner, M.D. for consultation on clinical issues in smoking cessation, and Edward Lichtenstein, Ph.D.

This book was a team effort. Jacqueline Varoli of LifeTime Media identified the need, developed the plan, and kept the project on target. Toni Goldfarb developed the text content with great diligence and care. Frances Jones put life, brevity, and wit into the prose. Celia Vimont and Karen Monaco from the American Lung Association identified resources from the Association's numerous materials on smoking and commented patiently on drafts of the text. Norman Edelman, M.D., senior medical consultant for the Lung Association, brought his knowledge and experience to the task of making sure the clinical and technical information was authoritative.

Index